THE MANAGEMENT OF CHRONIC ILLNESS

To Charles

THE MANAGEMENT OF CHRONIC ILLNESS

Patient and Doctor Perspectives on Parkinson's Disease

RUTH PINDER

MACMILLAN
PRESS

First published 1990

Published by
THE MACMILLAN PRESS LTD
Houndmills, Basingstoke, Hampshire RG21 2XS
and London
Companies and representatives
throughout the world

Filmset by Wearside Tradespools,
Fulwell, Sunderland

Printed in Hong Kong

British Library Cataloguing in Publication Data
Pinder, Ruth
The management of chronic illness.
1. Man. Parkinson's disease
I. Title
616.833
ISBN 0–333–48999–3
ISBN 0–333–49000–2 (pbk)

Contents

Foreword by Christopher Ashton   viii

Preface   x

Chapter 1: INTRODUCTION   1
Uncertainty and the patient–doctor relationship   1
Background   4
A note on the study   7
P.D.: Facts and figures   8

Chapter 2: EXPLAINING WHAT TO EXPECT: BELIEFS AND ROUTINES   11
Introduction   11
A spectrum of views   12
Routines and innovations   19
Summary and comment   23

Chapter 3: UNDERSTANDING THE IMPLICATIONS: KNOWLEDGE AS A RESOURCE?   25
Introduction   25
Information: friend or foe?   26
The role of the GP   34
Summary and comment   38

Chapter 4: THE DRUG REGIMEN: 'WE CAN TREAT IT'   41
Introduction   41
Rationale and side-effects   41
Something tangible on offer   46
Medical management or shared management?   48
Summary and comment   52

Chapter 5: THE HONEYMOON PERIOD—AND AFTER 54
   Introduction 54
   Misunderstandings and understandings 55
   Being on tablets 57
   Room for manoeuvre or playing it by the book? 59
   Patients' views of their GPs 63
   Summary and comment 66

Chapter 6: DETACHMENT OR EMPATHY? 68
   Introduction 68
   Down to basics: progression, incurability and 'the P.D. face' 69
   Exploring fears and anxieties 71
   Listening, and just being there 75
   Summary and comment 81

Chapter 7: CONTROLLING THE UNCONTROLLABLE: MAKING SENSE OF LIVING WITH P.D. 83
   Introduction 83
   Identity under threat 84
   In search of control 86
   Making a pact with P.D. 89
   How much can the GP offer? 91
   Summary and comment 95

Chapter 8: CONCLUSIONS: PATIENT AND DOCTOR— MATCH AND MISMATCH 97
   Introduction 97
   The study and its broader context 99
   Casting a wider net 100
   Match and mismatch 103
   Recommendations 109

Chapter 9: DOING RESEARCH: MORE THAN AN AFTER-THOUGHT 112
   Introduction 112
   Setting the scene 114
   Finding my patients and obtaining accounts 115
   GPs: An entry into a different world 118
   And after . . . 120
   Studying the powerless and the powerful 120

Appendix 1: PATIENT PROFILE 127

Appendix 2: DOCTOR PROFILE 129

References 130

Index 135

Foreword

It has often been stated that the care of a patient with a chronic illness should be based upon a close, effective relationship between patient and doctor. This relationship is of fundamental importance in determining how the patient experiences, manages and copes with his or her condition.

Using the model of Parkinson's Disease, Dr Pinder's research attempts to study and understand what it is that constitutes this fundamental, effective relationship. It was inspired by the lack of substantive emphasis and guidance on this aspect of care. Even in general practice, there has been, I believe, an emphasis on those aspects of the management of chronic illness which are most easily measured and have more to do with the structure than the content of care.

Dr Pinder has shown that understanding the doctor–patient relationship over the course of a progressive disabling illness such as Parkinson's Disease requires a departure from familiar models of medical research. To start with, I did not believe that an approach using such small numbers would have anything useful to contribute. It sounded anecdotal. In the light of her arguments, however, I have come to see things very differently. Not only is this a thoroughly systematic piece of research, fully as rigorous and demanding as the tradition in which I have been trained; it has yielded rich insights into the way patients and doctors manage a chronic illness from which the reader may gain considerable inspiration.

For the general practitioner the value of this work is twofold. First, in comparing and contrasting patients' views and feelings about various aspects of their illness, this research fosters a deeper understanding of the breadth of reaction to chronic illness. Second, all doctors will be able to identify with some of the attitudes expressed by the 18 general practitioners in this study. Reading the drafts of this book, I found that I often agreed with Dr Pinder's assessment of these attitudes, sometimes had to struggle to understand her critiques and occasionally protested loudly against them. The experience was always rewarding and the seeds of self-appraisal were planted.

Dr Pinder's achievement has been to identify from nine hundred pages of transcripted interviews certain attitudes, themes and concepts which further our understanding of the doctor–patient relationship over the course of a chronic illness.

I hope that these attitudes, themes and concepts are received by a wide audience, are understood, discussed, criticized and developed: they deserve to be.

July, 1989

Dr Christopher Ashton
Practising Family Practitioner,
Sutton Coldfield

Preface

'Why us? Why Parkinson's patients?' asked Mrs Unwin. It was a good question. The idea for this study arose from an interest in whether and, if so, to what extent, coming to terms with a debilitating illness was helped or hindered by patients' relationships with their GPs. That there might be two sides to this question was suggested by my husband's varied experiences with GPs at and after the onset of multiple sclerosis and, subsequently, by experience of others with M.S. At the time Parkinson's Disease seemed to have sufficient in common with M.S., while being interestingly different, to form the basis of a useful study.

I set out to study communication but soon found that I had to take a step back. It was necessary to consider first what both patient and doctor thought should and did happen between them. If, as is generally acknowledged, the presence of a caring, understanding and knowledgeable GP may make a great difference to the way patients experience and manage chronic illness, it is vitally important to understand what it is that makes for a satisfactory relationship, one that will be voluntarily sustained over time. It is this issue—communication in its widest sense—that the book seeks to address.

It reports on a research project conducted with a group of people with Parkinson's Disease (hereafter referred to as P.D. in the non-verbatim parts of the text) and a separate group of GPs, most of whom had had experience of P.D. patients. As the research shows, the experience and handling of the uncertainties inherent in chronic illness are the keys to the idea of satisfactory encounters between the two.

Doing the research for the book has left a lasting impression. I learned much from the patients who talked with me. I both knew, and in many ways did not know, what having P.D. was like. Pain and distress were evident and, trite as it may sound, so also was the sheer tenacity and courage patients showed in carrying on with life—some with, and others without, the support of their GP. It was, moreover, salutary to discover perfectly rational and intelligent patients who did not want to know 'the truth' about Parkinson's. My liberal ideas on the subject underwent a quiet sea-change.

I have explored the responses of patients and doctors to one particular condition, P.D. Yet it will be apparent that many of the thoughts and feelings expressed in this book could readily be applied to those with other chronic illnesses. But for the label, this could be patients speaking who have diabetes or rheumatoid arthritis. I believe GPs will also find similarities between their approach to P.D. patients and those suffering from the many other complaints with which they deal in their daily surgeries. This is a book as much about the universals as the particularities of people's responses to pain.

Despite initial apprehensions, interviewing GPs was a thoroughly enjoyable experience. Meeting them on a researcher–researched basis rather than in my normal capacity as a patient allowed me to see them as human beings, with the same strengths and frailties as others. This is not an anti-doctor book, and I hope that my comments will not be read in that light. In so far as I have been critical, this represents a plea for greater understanding in those areas where understanding may be most difficult to achieve. I hope that the findings will make a constructive contribution towards generating fresh thinking about general practice in the management of chronic illness.

Although I interviewed patients first, I have arranged the chapters so that doctors' accounts precede those of patients. The emphasis I wanted to achieve was: this is how GPs think about P.D. and communicating with their P.D. patients, but *this* is how patients see it. An appreciation of how *both* patient *and* doctor see the issues is the passport to a fuller understanding between them.

Chapter 1 introduces the concept of uncertainty, relates it to communication in the patient–doctor relationship and indicates where this study may extend our understanding. A brief note on the research design follows, and the chapter concludes with a short description of P.D., its incidence, prevalence and treatment.

The following chapters may most usefully be read in pairs, as a dialogue. Thus, Chapter 2 looks at the way GPs think about giving information to patients, while Chapter 3 traces patients' experience of coming to understand the illness and their own GPs' response to their struggles. Chapters 4 and 5 explore the two parties' views on handling information and sharing responsibility for the daily management of the drug treatment. Chapters 6 and 7 examine what the illness means to patients and how doctors and patients see the role of the GP in helping patients to come to terms with P.D. Chapter 8 draws these views and experiences together, looks at the broader implications for patient–doctor relationships in managing P.D. as well as other chronic illnesses, and suggests improvements in the education and training of GPs. The concluding chapter explores how the research was conducted and how my particular approach illuminates our understanding of the issues.

There are many people to thank for their support, particularly the Parkinson's Disease Society, which commissioned the research on which this book is based. The enthusiasm of the Society's Welfare Director, Mary Baker, often sustained me in writing this manuscript. I owe a special debt to my stalwart band of advisory readers. Dr Marie Oxtoby, Dr Christopher Ashton, Dr Roger Grimshaw and Judith Monks helped me to improve earlier drafts of this manuscript. John Morley OBE coaxed me to write tolerably crisp prose; and Dr Anna Wynne constantly encouraged me to scrutinize and broaden my ideas while alerting me to the nuances of a turn of phrase. Many of their suggestions have found their way into this text. Any errors or shortcomings are my responsibility alone. My thanks also go to my editor, David Grist; to Caroline Alexander for typing the text; and to Unwin Hyman for permission to reproduce passages from a chapter 'Striking balances: living with Parkinson's Disease' in Anderson and Bury's collection of studies on chronic illness. Above all, I want to thank the patients and GPs who generously gave their time and allowed me to share some of their thoughts and experiences. This book belongs to them.

London, January 1990   R.P.

1
Introduction

UNCERTAINTY AND THE PATIENT–DOCTOR RELATIONSHIP

Uncertainty about the future is the most fundamental and obvious aspect of the human condition. No one can predict accurately what is going to happen. We are constantly confronted by events which strain our precarious hold on certainty. Yet we act, most of the time, as though the world was orderly and predictable. We routinely go about our business as if uncertainty was not a problem in a world which is constantly throwing us askew. We make plans in the confident assurance that by and large they are likely to materialize. Indeed not to do so would be to abandon the whole precarious edifice upon which we construct our lives. Social life would be impossible without such assumptions of orderliness and predictability. By maintaining this 'as if' principle we assure ourselves of our place in the world and assert its continuity.

However, chronic illness, like other life crises, fractures this sense of coherence of the world (Bury, 1982; Charmaz, 1983). It is an assault on one's identity. The continuity of past, present and future is broken. Disorder is not a situation we can tolerate for long without making strenuous efforts to reduce it. To state that people need a certain amount of order in their lives is to state the obvious, but the struggle to impose order is absolutely fundamental to our personal and social survival. Murphy (1987, p. 29), himself progressively disabled with a spinal tumour, has eloquently described the problem:

> . . . it is an empirical fact that the mind seeks to impose systems of some kind of order upon all it surveys. It is a property of all peoples and all cultures. . . . We look for order because it makes predictability possible, and we seek predictability to avoid danger in an essentially perilous world. . . . Whether or not our structured images of the world around us correspond to an external reality, the predication of an order is necessary for intelligent creatures. It allows us to operate in a cockeyed world and to find meanings for our actions and lives in a milieu utterly devoid of absolute meanings.

To order life is also to make sense of what goes on, particularly with other people. To do so, we take a certain amount for granted and assume

1

that others share broadly similar views to our own. In practice, of course, different groups share different ideas about the world, a difference that becomes important when considering the special position held by doctors in our society. With the onset of illness, patients must meet members of a profession who may have different ideas and beliefs from themselves. It can no longer be taken for granted that the two coincide. This has crucial implications for communication. Patients and doctors need to make sense of what they are saying to one another. In turn, these interpretations—or perspectives—determine how patients and doctors view the relationship, what to expect from it, and in a very real sense what transpires within it. Barnlund (1976) reminds us:

> It is tempting in the daily clash of words to forget that it is the perceived world—not the real world—that we talk about, argue about, laugh about, cry about. It is not scalpels and crosses and bedpans that regulate human affairs, but how people construe them that determines what they will think, how they will feel, and what they will do about them.

However, the patient–doctor relationship in a chronic illness such as P.D. is a special case. Like chronic illness itself, it is often lengthy and unpredictable. It presents both patient and doctor with many problems, which include physical, practical, social and psychological difficulties. Above all, P.D. raises in acute form the problem of uncertainty for the two parties.

The basic issues stem from the same source: the difficulties of diagnosing the condition; the unpredictability of the way the illness may develop; and the variable effects and loss of effectiveness over time of the current drug regimen for any one patient. But the experience and management of P.D. gives rise to other uncertainties which are quite different for patient and doctor. I suggest that it is the way these non-medical uncertainties are differently perceived and handled by both parties which has critical implications for developing and sustaining a framework within which communication may flourish.

For the patient, uncertainty about the diagnosis, once resolved, leads to uncertainties as to what the label means, what course the illness will take, what to expect and when, which in turn may cause anxiety and distress. The ability to manage everyday living may no longer be taken for granted. Assumptions about sustaining roles within the family or at work are brought into question. Most importantly, the uncertainties of chronic illness raise profound human concerns, such as loss, and fears of dependence and of becoming what is unpleasantly termed 'a vegetable' in a culture which values self-reliance and economic and physical independence. The need to resolve the question 'What am I to make of life now that this has happened to me?' is always present. Uncertainty and its accompaniments—anxiety, fear and distress—are first-hand experiences for patients. They directly affect their lives.

For GPs uncertainties are different, but no less important. Doctors are faced with questions of how much to tell, when and to whom about the illness and the difficulties and limitations of the treatment. They must decide how much responsibility to delegate to patients, and how far to address patients' urgent need to find meaning in their new lives as P.D. patients. Most difficult of all, they must determine the nature and extent of their professional commitment to sharing patients' fundamental concerns when strictly medical solutions are comparatively short-term and partial. These areas of general practice are ill-defined and tend to highlight doctors' own personal anxieties and feelings of inadequacy and helplessness.

While the uncertainties are different, neither patient nor doctor can carry on unless they are, to some extent, managed. Both parties develop strategies and routines—shorthand ways of thinking which *become* routine—to do so. However, as the research shows, managing uncertainty means different things to patient and doctor. Patients are concerned with allowing in—with adjusting to what the illness means for their own lives and for those close to them. This is a new experience for patients. The strategies are partly techniques developed in response to the particular demands of the illness and its treatment and partly reflect an outlook on life generally.

Doctors, by contrast, are more concerned with shielding out—protecting patients from the impact of potentially distressing information, and themselves from feeling frustrated or inadequate in the face of human suffering. However, these are not new experiences for GPs. Routines are developed as a way of 'doing medicine' and are likely to be applied to many other conditions they face daily in their surgeries. A patient's illness is a doctor's work, an obvious point which is often overlooked.

This book explores how the different uncertainties of both parties and the way they are managed may both cause and be the result of difficulties in the patient–doctor relationship. Uncertainty may both result *in* miscommunication, with patient and doctor engaged in seemingly incompatible activities, and itself be the result *of* miscommunication, what is seen to be happening in the relationship leading to frustration or distress. Therefore, we are dealing both with possible miscommunication—actual encounters may go awry—and with communication breakdown—there may be no physical communication at all. Patients can choose whether or not to consult their own GPs.

I shall further examine how, in the face of uncertainty, patients and GPs may develop different ideas of managing the same illness, and the consequences of this for interaction between them. By exploring their different perspectives, I intend to highlight ways in which these may be brought closer together and communication improved. I believe that if doctors are able positively and openly to address the ways that patients, and they themselves, experience and try to handle uncertainty, the whole relationship may be greatly enhanced. It is only through such an understanding that GPs may judge the extent to which they are giving a satisfactory and relevant service.

There are many possible points during the course of a patient's illness where the two parties' concerns may meet. However, I have deliberately avoided dealing with the diagnosis. While the quest for certainty had often started for patients well before this, and difficulty in diagnosis was the problem most readily mentioned by GPs, I wanted to concentrate on the much more difficult area of on-going management of the illness. For patients, what happened after the diagnosis was often as important as receiving the label in the first place. By emphasizing this post-diagnostic period, I am able to focus on the continuing nature of patient–doctor communication over a range of issues.

I have chosen to explore three areas: explaining and coming to understand what to expect of the illness; managing the drug regimen; and the provision of, and need for, social and psychological support. These were areas identified by patients in the study as being most important in assessing the helpfulness and relevance of their GP and, as the research also demonstrates, proved to be more difficult for doctors than they at first anticipated.

BACKGROUND

This section is mainly for social scientists and those particularly interested in the study's wider context. The general reader may pick up the story on p. 7 with 'A Note on the Study'. There is a vast literature on the doctor–patient relationship and doctor–patient communication. However, as overviews of some of the major writings and trends make plain (see, for example, Hauser, 1981; Pendleton and Hasler, 1983; Morgan *et al.*, 1985), they focus on issues such as class, age, educational background, gender, the 'competence gap', the dominance of the biomedical approach to communication and the inequality in status between patient and doctor. While these are important, I believe that the status of patienthood, or rather the uncertainty which characterizes this particular type of patienthood, transcends these concerns. I depart from these writings, therefore, in five important respects.

First, I am concerned to analyse the relationship between patient and general practitioner. The many studies which have examined doctor–patient communication have largely been between chronically ill patients and hospital physicians (see, for example, Davis, 1963; West, 1976; Darling, 1979; Speedling, 1982). The GP is mentioned only tangentially, and mostly negatively, as having inadequate knowledge of the condition in question.

Second, studies which have analysed patient–GP communication have concentrated on the consultation itself, where communication is tied to a particular place and time (see, for instance, Byrne and Long, 1976; Tuckett *et al.*, 1985). My concern here is not with what 'actually' happened but the broader question of patients' and GPs' respective ideas about managing the uncertainties which are raised with the onset of P.D.

Third, there have been relatively few attempts to explore the work of GPs in relation to specific patient groups or illness conditions—with the exception of Maguire's work on GPs and cancer patients (1984, 1985) and the work of Still and Todd (1986) on GPs and the terminally ill. P.D. may well provide a model for the study of other chronic illnesses which increasingly form part of a GP's caseload.

Fourth, we have not often had the chance of seeing how communication looks from the viewpoints of both patient and doctor. Research which considers how these two perspectives may match or mismatch in the management of a difficult chronic illness has been largely ignored by others (with the notable exception of the case studies described by Kleinman, 1988).

Fifth, and most importantly, I am exploring a comparatively neglected area: that of the management of uncertainty as a key concept in the patient–doctor relationship. Calnan (1984) has suggested that it is only in cases where the patient becomes responsible for his/her treatment, or becomes well-informed—characteristics of the chronically ill—that the issue of uncertainty is important. He did not develop the point. Given the anxieties and distress which often accompany P.D., we need to understand how they are experienced and handled.

The limited work on the management of uncertainty which has been done has largely concerned the training of medical students and has been applied to hospital physicians rather than GPs (Fox, 1957, 1959, 1980). She examined how doctors are trained to handle three types of uncertainty: inadequate mastery of the available medical knowledge; the limitations of medical knowledge itself; and, most importantly, the difficulties of distinguishing between the two. However, Atkinson (1984) suggests that such a view is too simplistic and glosses over important distinctions. Doubt, puzzlement or bewilderment, he argues, are 'a far cry from . . . the sort of generalized cultural crisis or *angst* which Fox also claims is linked to such "uncertainty"'.

I, too, am concerned with different orders of uncertainty. However, Atkinson's work was concerned with hospital training, where doctors are generally protected from experiencing undue uncertainty by the close-knit hospital structure, by an emphasis on knowledge as a discrete set of facts to be learned, or not, and by the concentration on acute rather than chronic illness. The situation in general practice is more diffuse. In analysing the patient–GP relationship in chronic illness, I believe that the concept of uncertainty has much to offer in explaining the way patients and their GPs perceive their differing worlds, so long as the different dimensions are scrupulously identified and uncertainty does not become the 'catch-all' notion Atkinson rightly criticizes.

The study of uncertainty as a controlling device in the physician–patient relationship is particularly important here (see Light, 1979). Davis's (1963) classic study of parents of children with polio found that clinical uncertainty was often used by doctors to defer having to give explanations about prognosis—a process he referred to as 'functional uncertainty' (Davis, 1960). This latter concept has been useful in explaining the practice of doctors withholding information, particularly at points of diagnosis and prognosis (see, for example, the works of Roth, 1963, and West, 1976).

McIntosh's (1977) seminal study of doctors' communication with cancer patients is most pertinent to this research. He describes the routines developed both by doctors to control uncertainty—typically by the non-disclosure of information, especially about prognosis—and by patients in trying to acquire information consistent with retaining hope. His study shows that the process of communicating information and acquiring understanding is much more complex and subtle than was previously thought.

McIntosh's study has been an inspiration and I am indebted to him for introducing me to the concept in the first place. This research extends his work in two ways. First, it explores the management of uncertainty in relation to information-giving, *and* to the difficult areas of providing emotional support and encouraging varying degrees of self-management in treatment. Second, it examines the way uncertainty is experienced and handled within the context of general practice. A relationship between patient and GP in chronic illness is quite unlike that between patient and physician in hospital.

For patients, the management of uncertainty has been discussed as part of a wider repertoire of 'coping' skills and is becoming increasingly well documented since the publication of Strauss and Glaser's (1975) innovative work on the subject (see, for instance, Speedling, 1982; Schneider and Conrad, 1983; Pinder, 1988; Robinson, 1988). It has been addressed as a focal issue in studies of rheumatoid arthritis (Wiener, 1975), cystic fibrosis (Waddell, 1982) and diabetes (Mason, 1985). But the way patients experience and manage uncertainty has not been directly linked to their ideas about communication with their GPs. Crucially, to the best of my knowledge, no study has examined the differing ways uncertainty is experienced and handled by both patient and GP over a range of issues which arise as a patient's illness unfolds, and their implications for the patient–doctor relationship. This book sets out to address this issue.

A NOTE ON THE STUDY

A more detailed discussion of the way the study was conducted, and some of the problems and broader issues it raised, are to be found in Chapter 9. Brief factual information about the patients and doctors studied is arranged in the Patient and Doctor Profiles in Appendices 1 and 2.

My concern is with ideas, feelings, interpretations and experience—not figures and measurements. This dictated the use of a qualitative approach, one which specifically lends itself to exploring ideas and experiences 'from the inside'. The research tools used reflected this approach. Multiple in-depth interviews which encouraged a free-ranging discussion of ideas about patients' experiences of the illness and their encounters with GPs were conducted with fifteen patients over an initial period of fifteen months. These were followed by single interviews, for a minimum of forty-five minutes, with a separate group of eighteen GPs, sixteen of whom had direct experience with P.D. patients. These took place over ten months, and focused on themes identified by patients as causing difficulties and distress. Further informal meetings with patients, and in three cases the widows of former patients, took place in the course of writing this book. Altogether these interviews yielded about one hundred hours of tape-recorded conversation and the transcriptions covered some nine hundred typed pages. These verbatim accounts form the evidence from which interpretations and conclusions are drawn. It should be noted that patients and doctors were all interviewed before the possibility of using fetal transplants became a public issue. The use of drugs formed the standard medical treatment.

I tried to classify patients into groups according to the perceived helpfulness or otherwise of their GPs. The limitations of reliance on global evaluations alone will be discussed further in Chapter 9. Although there were patients at both extremes who found their GPs 'very helpful' or 'unhelpful'—evaluations which held across a range of issues—there was a mixed group who found their GPs supportive about some issues but not others. Critically, patients' reactions changed over time. I have, therefore, only grouped patients informally in the text for this purpose.

When I considered the strategies patients developed to understand what the illness and drug regimen meant for their lives, certain distinctions did emerge. However, these were not consistent across a range of other responses, such as sharing treatment decisions, and they bore little relation to the more general problem of coming to terms with the illness itself. I have drawn distinctions where they made a useful contribution to the analysis.

Equally, I have not classified doctors in any formal way. As I am exploring several different issues about communication, and differing orientations within each, only the most general descriptive term does justice to the complexity of their responses—namely, the flexibility or otherwise with which GPs approached the task of communicating with their patients. I have used this term descriptively as far as possible, as one which broadly represented doctors' policies. No moral judgement is intended. Although doctors' responses did differ—particularly in respect of conveying information about the illness—there were also considerable areas of overlap. I have brought out the similarities and differences where these occurred in the text.

To preserve anonymity, I have referred to patients and doctors in the text by pseudonyms chosen at random. Any similarity to real people bearing the same name is purely fortuitous. My initial policy of using initials and numbers was uncomfortably impersonal. The intention is that each patient and doctor will recognize him/herself but will otherwise be unidentifiable. I have referred to place names and other personal details, such as hospitals attended, as 'X', etc. The names of patients' own GPs have been similarly camouflaged.

It was impossible to give everyone an equal voice. Some patients and doctors talked more fluently and illustrated particular points more vividly than others. Moreover, the wealth of data collected cannot be confined within a single volume. Nevertheless, I have tried to give everyone a hearing and to reproduce, as faithfully as possible, the wishes and intentions of the patients and doctors as expressed in the tapes. Their stories form the substance of this book.

P.D.: FACTS AND FIGURES

While many of the findings in this study have implications for other chronic conditions, this book is specifically about P.D. Describing what P.D. is has been largely the province of the medical profession ever since its clinical manifestations were first outlined by Dr James Parkinson in 1817. Emphasis has been on questions of differential diagnosis, medical management, discussion of possible breakthroughs in treatment and, latterly, epidemiology. As this is one side of the coin with which GPs work, it is important to bear such definitions in mind, while arguing later for an alternative conceptualization.

P.D. is an incurable, degenerative disease of the nervous system, the cause of which remains unknown. The onset of the illness is gradual. Many early symptoms, such as vague aches and pains, fatigue, slightly impaired speech or difficulty in controlling fine movements of the hands, often pass unnoticed and are difficult to diagnose. Its effects also vary considerably as between individuals. The classic triad of symptoms—tremor, rigidity and slowness of movement—may only arise later, and some patients may be affected by one more than another. As the illness progresses, other symptoms, such as chronic fatigue, early morning slowness of movement, deterioration in clarity and volume of speech, stooping gait, giddy turns, or episodes of freezing or start-hesitation, may occur, again affecting some patients but not others. Stern and Lees (1982) note: 'Each patient is a law unto himself.'

P.D. is one of the most common disabling neurological conditions after stroke (Godwin-Austen and Hildick-Smith, 1982). The Office of Health Economics (1974) study suggested that: 'About two-thirds of those who suffer from it for ten years become very dependent on physical assistance from others during that period.'

Until recently, P.D. was said to affect one person per thousand population. The Royal College of Physicians (1986) study suggests that the figure may be twice this, with some 112 000 people having the illness in the UK, as opposed to earlier estimates of 60 000–80 000 (Office of Health Economics, 1974). Even these figures may underestimate the prevalence of P.D. Misdiagnosis, and the unwillingness of people to consult their doctors with what may be mild symptoms, are thought to be common.

Many studies show that the prevalence of P.D. rises sharply with age (Hildick-Smith, 1980). Some authors suggest a peak at about seventy-five years, declining thereafter (Schoenberg, 1986), but Mutch *et al.* (1986) suggest a much later point in the ninth decade. As P.D. more commonly occurs during later life, the increasing number of those aged over eighty-five in the population has important implications for the scope of future general practice (O.P.C.S. Monitor, 1986). The average GP may need to care for between three and five known P.D. patients per practice (Thompson, 1987), who are likely to present complex management problems.

Prior to the advent of levodopa therapy, there was little effective treatment for P.D. The anticholinergic drugs were the main drugs of choice, and are still used today in the early stages of treatment. However, the discovery of dopamine deficiency in the brain in the early 1960s led to the production of high-dose oral levodopa treatment in 1967. Like insulin, it is a replacement therapy, not a cure. It cannot halt the underlying progression of the disease.

Early enthusiasm about its discovery has diminished with the appearance of serious side-effects in patients treated over time. These may include involuntary writhing movements, confusion or memory disturbance, and sudden, unpredictable swings from 'on' to 'off', the severity of which have been accentuated by levodopa (Marsden and Parkes, 1976; Marsden *et al.*, 1982).

Nevertheless, there have been substantial improvements since 1967. The administration of levodopa is now combined with additives, and the decarboxylase inhibitors Sinemet and Madopar form the basic treatment for the illness. Other drugs designed to mimic the effects of levodopa, such as Bromocriptine (Parlodel), have been found helpful, and work is currently being done to try and modify the severity and duration of that most refractory side-effect, the 'on'/'off' syndrome (Stibe *et al.*, 1988). The preliminary results of a recent study have shown that the early administration of deprenyl (Selegiline) prolongs the period before the severity of disability necessitates the initiation of levodopa therapy (The Parkinson Study Group, 1989).

Thus, while the benefits of the drugs have been impressive, giving in many cases a 'honeymoon period' of between two and five years in the early stages of the illness, and, with the benefit of deprenyl, perhaps longer in future, where symptoms may be well controlled, their long-term use remains highly problematic. Some clinicians consider that the future lies less in discovering a 'better DOPA' than in finding the underlying mechanism(s) of the loss of dopamine cells in the brain (Barbeau, 1981). In these circumstances the excitement raised by the transplantation of brain cells from aborted fetuses into the brains of a few P.D. patients in 1988 was understandable. Long-term evaluation of the technique is, of course, essential before any claims as to its possible benefits may be made. However, such developments raise the wider issue of the position of the chronically ill at the very frontiers of scientific knowledge. Chronically ill patients are often the true experimenters.

The facts—or the lack of them—seem to have a taken-for-grantedness about them, as technical problems which, with further application, will be resolved in due season. Reading the literature one experiences, as a lay person, a curious sense of detachment from those suffering the consequences of such an illness. Where is the human face in these descriptions? This is the interface at which GPs work. For GPs to help patients, facts and figures must become personalized. The GP is in a unique position, having to mediate between the world of facts and their translation as a service to patients. This book is concerned both with GPs' views of the application of this kind of certainty-amidst-uncertainty and with highlighting a perspective which is frequently ignored: the patient's viewpoint. At stake are the ways in which patients and doctors experience the uncertainties to which the facts give rise and, in turn, how these may affect building a caring, supportive patient–doctor relationship.

2
Explaining What to Expect: Beliefs and Routines

'It's not difficult to tell a patient that they've got Parkinson's—not that they've got Parkinson's—but what it actually means.'

INTRODUCTION

Once a diagnosis has been made, GPs are faced with further uncertainties, both clinically and personally. Chapter 1 described the variability of the prognosis of the illness in any one patient and the difficulties of predicting its course with any accuracy. However, doctors do know the parameters of the disease, from the best to the worst case, knowledge which few patients are likely to possess at the outset. As Davis (1963, p. 49) has pointed out: 'The possibility of important uncertainty factors . . . is not the same thing as total ignorance of the probabilities.'

Potentially more difficult to handle are the uncertainties involved in gauging how much patients want to know of the implications and when. There is a wealth of evidence to show that partial disclosure or non-disclosure of information, where it is wanted, bewilders and frustrates patients' attempts to understand (see, for example, Power and Sax (1978); Locker (1983); Quine and Pahl (1986)). Conversely, things said cannot be unsaid if the situation is misjudged. However, studies have tended to stress the difficulties for patients in the former situation. The delicate task of timing disclosure of information and managing patients who are not ready to know has received less attention.

GPs have no easily verifiable way of knowing whether explanations given to, or withheld from, patients are what patients want, or, if told 'the truth', how patients will respond. Judgements have to be made. The questions are how are they made, what purposes do they serve and, most importantly, what are their likely effects on communication between patient and doctor?

Every helping profession routinely adopts socially agreed ways of processing people (Prottas, 1979; Cantley and Hunter, 1985). Like every-

11

one else, doctors are engaged in making their environment meaningful. The people to be 'processed' must be sorted into easily recognized categories if orderly decision-making is to occur. Doctors then develop routines to help them work more efficiently. My argument is that while the use of judgements and routines may reduce *doctors'* uncertainties, they also have consequences for communication which may or may not be helpful to patients.

This chapter explores how GPs in the study responded to the question of explaining what to expect. I shall examine how doctors placed patients into varying categories and developed routines with which to handle uncertainty. I suggest that where such beliefs and routines remained unquestioned, decision-making was simplified, reducing the anxiety which might arise if each case was treated individually. Conversely, where beliefs were more flexible and allowed for greater openness, GPs were attuned to patients' individual needs. Frankness itself reduced ambiguity.

GPs' beliefs and routines varied according to whether they preferred to adopt mainly closed, mixed or mainly open responses. Beliefs about patients often occurred in clusters. Some, however, featured more prominently than others in doctors' accounts and merit particular attention— namely, those relating to age, intelligence and educational background, and the broader judgement of 'what patients can cope with'.

A SPECTRUM OF VIEWS

The Question of Age: *'Disability in ten years is much less important to an older person than to a younger one'*

Some doctors referred to age as determining what should be explained. Dr Black and Dr Wilkinson thought that with age the onset of handicapping illness was a much less upsetting experience. Dr Wilkinson said of his P.D. patients: 'I think they more or less regard it as part of the ageing process. They're not *unduly* distressed by the whole thing.'

Dr Naughton contrasted P.D. with multiple sclerosis: 'Parkinson's Disease is rarely that distressing . . . M.S. tends to be in younger people. They tend to suffer more and longer. I've got two families with severely handicapped people with M.S. Their lives are wretched and the lives of everyone around them are wretched.' It was not that GPs were unsympathetic with their P.D. patients. No GP in the study was insensitive or unfeeling towards those with the disease. Rather, their sympathies were particularly engaged with those who became disabled before their lives had had a chance to flower. Yet, in making this distinction, Dr Naughton indicated that there were important implications for patient–doctor communication:

I find around here that my elderly people don't want to know a great deal about it and I think that's right. I don't see it as an area where a huge amount of communicating has to be done. . . . These people . . . have all been over sixty, in their seventies or eighties and some nineties. I've never made a diagnosis in someone under seventy. So I haven't seen it as an issue that involved a lot of doctor–patient interaction.

Doctors did not consider that the nuances involved in gauging what details to explain about the illness and when to convey them were so necessary for older patients. Such judgements were reserved for those in younger age groups.

GPs using Dr Naughton's line of reasoning relied on everyday experience in managing this potentially difficult area of communication. The confidence with which they made their assertions indicated that doctors had little doubt about their validity, although beliefs were largely untested and unquestioned. Communication was simplified and detailed discussion about what to expect which might be distressing was avoided.

Several doctors distinguished those patients born before World War I from 'younger and more articulate patients', as having 'less highly developed expectations . . . being less questioning because they respect doctors more' and as being content to be told what to do rather than wishing to share in decision-making. Dr Perlmann explained:

A lot of old people seem to prefer the doctor saying 'this is the case' and doesn't explore five different possibilities and then say 'which one do you think is reasonable?' They find that very difficult to cope with. It's not their concept of what a doctor does. As we all get older maybe our views and those of Parkinson's patients will change.

Again implicit in doctors' accounts were references to the 'obviousness' of experience. Yet this rarely seemed to be put to the test. Confidence in subjective assessment poses a paradox in a profession which respects the value of science and the requirements of scientific proof. However, students learn to value clinical experience (as opposed to the application of theoretical knowledge) early in their medical careers (Knafl and Burkett, 1978). Dr Fleming illustrated the tension between these two imperatives. Initially he accounted for his beliefs about age which were similar to those of the doctors cited above, by reference to experience. Yet he was beginning to question himself. He ventured tentatively over the 'phone:

I don't know, it's an attitude, experience. It must be experience, maybe very limited. It *does* avoid uncertainty. It *also* depends on how articulate patients are. For a patient who's highly articulate you'd feel under great pressure to provide explanations and supply them with information . . . though the need for information may be just the same for someone who's not articulate. . . .

In questioning his own views he discovered, to his surprise, that both he and his colleagues were, as he put it, 'guilty of ageism'. When one assumption was questioned, he changed tack and produced an alternative working hypothesis only to find that equally inadequate. When he was stripped of the certainty which reliance on such beliefs provided, he found he had to rethink his working philosophy. It was not always a comfortable process, as other GPs in the study indicated.

Such views on ageing may reflect the stereotypes which abound in our culture, where the elderly are variously seen as incompetent, socially irrelevant and subject to a wide range of imperfections, including ill-health. However, more recent evidence, does not support the view that disability and age are so highly correlated (Victor, 1987; Freer, 1988). Fennell *et al.* (1988), reviewing the literature on older women and illness, concluded that ill-health was far from being a universal accompaniment of old age.

It seemed that GPs were no more able to resist absorbing stereotypes than others. Fear of ageing is deeply embedded in Western culture. Simone de Beauvoir (1970) noted: 'Nothing should be more expected than old age; nothing is more unforeseen.' She quotes (p. 10) from Proust: '"Of all realities [old age] is perhaps that of which we retain a purely abstract notion longest in our lives"'. By treating old age as a category, these GPs may also have found a way of handling their own personal fears and anxieties. Moreover, the development of routine assumptions about the old simplified management. It absolved doctors from having to make potentially anxiety-laden decisions about what to convey to their older P.D. patients. Detailed explanations about what to expect were not necessary.

By contrast, other doctors minimized ambiguity in decision-making by adopting more open, flexible policies towards giving information. The use of broad categories such as age did not determine what was seen as appropriate to explain. Dr Leadbrough, for instance, compared P.D. patients with others who might similarly be thought of as less interested in and competent to handle explanations about what to expect:

> I think the whole time you've got to *try* and treat people as individuals. It's easier said than done. You know there are lots of reasons for not telling people things at different ages. You could say the same thing of children, that they're incompetent. I don't necessarily feel that because they're senile dements that they shouldn't have as much of a sporting chance of information as anyone else.

She recognized the role of beliefs in affecting decisions about explaining and the difficulties of adhering to a model of treating the whole person. The ideology of individualized care was often not compatible with such beliefs. Nevertheless, she felt that by sharing information, patients could cope with more than expected by her peers. Given a presumption of openness towards patients, the anxiety surrounding any decision as to whether to tell patients or not did not arise. The question, as we shall see, was one of trying to pace information according to the perceived needs of the patient. It seemed that these doctors had a counselling approach and had developed special skills in empathy which enabled such sensitive tailoring to individual needs to take place—a picture which emerges with particular clarity in Chapter 6.

A Preference for the Intelligent Patient: *'One of the constraints is undoubtedly the intelligence or educational attainment of the person you're dealing with'*

Judgements about patients' intelligence and educational background—and more generally about what patients could cope with—were also important in managing uncertainty and in determining what was considered appropriate to communicate.

The issue initially seemed fairly clear-cut for Dr Quinn. He was confident of the reliability of his judgements. He said of one of his patients:

> I think she had rather a low IQ and I don't think she asked any questions about the illness. Of course I think it's a different kettle of fish if someone's educated, say someone from a different class who contracted the disease. They'd want to know everything about it. . . . You know the strata of your patients, whether they're intelligent or educated. I think it differs an awful lot. I'm trying to think of the word—literate. The more *literate* patients are the more questions they ask, obviously.

Intelligence and literacy were unquestionably associated in his mind with a desire to know all the facts, however dire their implications.

However, a poignant situation had arisen. Dr Quinn's long-held belief in the desirability of a fairly closed approach to the disclosure of information had been visibly shaken following the diagnosis of his wife's breast cancer. His peers' failure to communicate effectively with the couple had left him bewildered and confused. He was unable to reconcile a lifetime's work as a GP with the frustration and anxiety caused by minimal explanations of what to expect in his personal situation. Putting his feelings into words was difficult for him. His talk was punctuated by stops, starts and hesitations:

> I know the problem is the transfer of information to the patient . . . and really it was amazing. Although I'd treated cancer all my years to have it happen in your family. You're really at a loss to find out about things. . . . It was a bit of a shock and I thought really we should have been told more at the hospital. Sister or someone should have told us what to do and how to get help. We had to root around.

His expectation that intelligence, not to mention membership of the same professional community, would produce explanations enabling him to understand what to expect had not materialized. There was a gulf between knowledge and understanding—between conveying the facts on the one hand and the more difficult task of facilitating understanding in patients on the other. They were not on the same cognitive level.

Other GPs who wanted to contain the situation more closely 'kept the information simple'. Dr Ogilvie eliminated 'the fine details of the illness unless the patient is particularly interested or quite intelligent and able to grasp complex disorders'. Some doctors stressed the need for repetition. However, remembering all the facts does not necessarily indicate understanding. People have to make sense of the facts according to what is important to them. Not everything that a doctor says has equivalent significance (Tuckett *et al.*, 1985). Moreover, the possibility that less articulate patients may still want to understand—a situation of some complexity and uncertainty—did not form part of the calculation. The very use of such judgements absolved GPs from having to make difficult decisions which might give rise to intense anxiety, as McIntosh (1977) found of the hospital physicians he studied. Ambiguity was minimized.

GPs with more varied views on the extent to which the implications of the illness could be conveyed in any detail agreed that explaining what to expect was difficult. Dr Black put the dilemmas very clearly:

> I make judgements based on my assessments of the patient's personality, his educational background and his intelligence and whether I think he's likely to be able to take it in and benefit from the information I give him really. Perhaps this is a bit patronizing and I don't know what right I've got to do that, but obviously one doesn't want to overload someone with technical terms which they can't possibly understand. At the same time, I don't want to leave people feeling frustrated and feeling they've not been told anything. To get it just right.

However, difficulties had to be managed if doctors were not to be paralysed by indecision. Work had to be accomplished. The question is the extent to which judgements allowed for the emergence of the patient as a person, with individual needs and expectations.

Several doctors in the study challenged their peers' judgements about what patients could cope with, some with hesitation and others with more confidence. Dr Smythe, for example, was not altogether comfortable about the possible outcome of changing his approach. He explained:

> Their social class doesn't come into it. But certainly their intelligence, their ability to manipulate the tablets they're taking and to actually understand what Parkinson's means. And we have a lot of illiterate patients round here and a lot of patients don't understand the term 'deterioration'. It's much harder to explain to them what it does mean and I think that can lead to frustration. But, on the other hand, those patients go away often more satisfied with less questioning of their problems. But yes, they get a poorer deal.

Like Dr Fleming, when he found one way of categorizing patients wanting, he rapidly substituted it with another: the less intelligent were easily satisfied and easier to please. Dr Richards was rather more assured. While claiming 'I don't think people remember an awful lot', he nevertheless felt able to adopt communication strategies that allowed for differences in people's levels of understanding:

I don't like using the word 'intelligence'. It's positively loaded. Perhaps I'd put it much more in terms of whether someone has an interest. You can pick up cues from people. Often I find people who are not so intelligent are nonetheless interested in what's going on and you can explain it in terms which mean something. I'm not particularly good at it, but I think you do pick up these things from people.

These GPs had more flexible views about their patients. Correspondingly, responses could be tailored to meet individual needs without provoking too much anxiety. Indeed, doctors needed to know what was happening in order to target their explanations sensitively and effectively. Sharing information—and its attendant uncertainties—was in itself liberating as we shall see in more detail later.

What Patients Can Cope with: *'Blinding them with science doesn't help. It really makes them more anxious and frustrated'*

The fear of distressing patients (and its assumed consequences) was also important in governing what doctors chose to say. Some doctors were anxious to limit opportunities for discussion. They thought that it was in the patient's best interests to be protected from the impact of any distressing information. Little information was necessary. The uncertainty of the clinical prognosis allowed Dr Victor, for example, to pursue a fairly closed policy towards information giving. Referring to one of his patients, he said:

If I *know* what the future's going to hold I'm happy to talk about it, but it's pointless making statements about an illness when you don't really know. . . . Parkinson's is such a chronic illness. If I'd told him in 1960 that he'd still be dribbling in 1986 how would it have helped? I think I'm as Irish as he is and probably just take things as they come. I do the best I can. I don't think I'd ever be terribly enthusiastic about trying to tell Parkinson's patients what the future holds, which is really not very good. . . . M.S. is a classic example. And if you tell everyone with M.S. that they're going to be bed-ridden it doesn't do them any good and it's probably not right. And I think Parkinson's is very much the same.

He assumed that patients did not want to know and therefore there was little point in worrying them unnecessarily. Although the prognosis was probably not good, he could not be categorical about this. The clinical uncertainty inherent in the prognosis supported this line of reasoning.

By contrast, other doctors assumed not only that patients wanted to know the truth, but also that they had a right to information about the illness and its prognosis. Dr Young, for instance, felt that 'being absolutely honest' with patients simplified decision-making and, moreover, ultimately enabled patients to cope better. She explained:

Some people say 'It's an awful illness and you don't want to frighten the patient too much', but I'm afraid I don't agree with that. I think if that's the illness they've got it's their right to have the information. You don't obviously say to the person 'You know you're going to be completely incapacitated', you don't floor a person with that, but you gradually get them used to the idea that it is deteriorating. Otherwise they're going to get terribly wound up about the fact that it isn't being fixed. . . . But if you don't give them any information, they can't come to terms with it and they can't organize their lives.

She thought that, with help, patients could cope. It was unfair to deprive them of knowledge which could help them to manage the illness. A policy of openness again had distinct advantages for these GPs. Dr Richards and Dr Young agreed that they did not have to worry about who was told what. It resolved uncertainties on that score.

Two GPs discovered that the question of protecting patients from distress was more complex than they had thought. Dr Miller and Dr Leadbrough recognized an equally important right *not* to know. Their views challenge the more liberal orthodoxy in which doctors are now being trained. For doctors accustomed to openness, this step backwards was a difficult one to take. Dr Miller had only recently recognized its importance in her work with the terminally ill. It caused her some initial disquiet until she felt comfortable with both positions. She commented:

I found that while I was usually trained in that everything's going to be the ideal death, there were some families in which some people wanted to know and some people didn't want to know, and that it wasn't necessarily right for me to say 'We must discuss this'.

Judgements had to be made on a more individual basis. Responses could not be standardized. Doctors needed to be guided by what Dr Ellis called 'the natural history of the patient' in deciding what information to convey and when.

Again these doctors were able to challenge the judgements of some of their colleagues. Dr Young said:

A lot of doctors are very wary of giving people bad news because they think somehow they're going to stop functioning, they're going to go out and sit and starve, or they're going to kill themselves. But mostly people don't. Mostly people come to terms with it. They may come to terms with it at different stages. I've been stunned by people's responses. All sorts of people who you would think would be very stoical kind of disintegrate on you and vice versa. . . . You can't really judge how people are going to react from how they carried on before.

In redefining her own approach she was, of course, relying on a different set of beliefs, which in turn were predicated on a different view of patients. She expected them to be distressed, both initially and at various times as the illness progressed, but not generally to collapse—a more dynamic view which avoided approaching patients with the 'set' of expectations identified by Verby *et al.* (1979) and Byrne and Long (1984) as a common pattern among GPs studied. Moreover, as other doctors discovered, uncertainties could be shared, defusing the situation. A more flexible policy towards communication entailed paying attention to cues from patients as to when they were ready to take on board further details. The question was one of sensitive timing, allowing patients to set the pace—not one of deciding whether or not to disclose information in the first place.

COMMENT

Some doctors' policies suggested that the use of broad judgements relating to age, intelligence and what patients could or could not cope with reduced the uncertainty involved in not knowing which patients to tell. Patients were told little or were given very simple explanations. But doctors' approaches differed. In this my findings support the earlier evidence of Comaroff (1976), who explored the varied policies of a group of GPs towards giving information about non-fatal illnesses to their patients. As we have seen, other GPs in this study had a more flexible approach. A wider range of alternative ways of explaining the facts was available. By being more open with patients, these GPs were not caught up in anxiety-making dilemmas of who should be told what. They relied on pointers from patients to alert them as to when and how much to disclose. They needed this information to ensure that they were on target. Explaining and helping patients to understand what to expect was a shared experience. Ambiguity was minimized.

The difficulties were perhaps greatest for those doctors who were aware of the complexities involved but found that reliance on simpler judgements was necessary if they were to cope. Their changing assumptions suggested that the management of uncertainty was not always so neatly resolved. Other devices had to be employed.

ROUTINES AND INNOVATIONS

'I'd say "I don't think that in the foreseeable future you will find your lifestyle's greatly changed, or find yourself greatly handicapped by Parkinson's"'

Doctors developed special routines to minimize the uncertainties of not knowing how patients might react to sensitive information. These included the use of optimism, particularly by stressing the variability of the prognosis and by spinning out time. Doctors also had policies about question responding or initiating.

The Value of Optimism

Most doctors wanted to stress the positive side of the illness, although the emphasis varied among doctors. The chief concern was for patients to retain hope and not worry unduly: patients who worried were likely to be difficult to manage. In addition, the use of optimism absolved GPs from having to confront their patients with the less pleasant aspects of the illness. The negative side of the coin was avoided where possible or, as Dr Ellis noted, 'played down' in the first instance.

Several doctors stressed the variability of the prognosis. They deliberately emphasized clinical uncertainty to encourage patients to see their own case in a more favourable light. Such terms as 'yours is a mild case' were frequently used. Dr Black, for instance, said of one of his patients:

> I put it that the progression's rather variable, that he wouldn't necessarily develop the symptoms, or if he did it might take many years. That many other things can happen in that time. . . . I tried to support him by saying that there were varying degrees of the illness and that this was a very mild one and that there were drugs to deal with it. That there was help we could give him.

As patients commonly consulted their GPs in the earlier stages of the illness, such an assessment was not unreasonable. Stressing the positive aspects of P.D. and concentrating on what could be done to 'control the illness' reduced anxieties all round. The situation, as Dr Wilkinson recalled telling one of his patients, 'wasn't as bad as she thought it was'.

Other doctors were similarly positive. Dr Fleming noted of a patient: 'I have painted an optimistic picture, perhaps an unduly optimistic picture, and I'm aware that in doing so it's *easier* for me to give good news than to give bad news.' The uncertainty which 'being realistic' might entail was minimized. Doctors wanted to spare patients (and themselves) as much distress and anxiety as possible. Dr Quinn was quite categorical on this point: 'I never paint a black picture about them [the chronic sick]. I'd always be optimistic.'

In their explanations, doctors encouraged their patients to take a long view of their illness. It could be years before patients might anticipate any appreciable degree of handicap. They urged patients to focus on the present. The fact that nothing serious was likely to happen immediately gave doctors room for manoeuvre. They stressed the 'near-normality' which could be achieved. The prospect of their patients having to face serious disability was relegated to some unspecified time in the distant future, so as to approximate people's general ideas about life expectancy. Dr Ogilvie's response provides a good illustration of this approach:

> He might ask 'What's going to happen to my life-span? Will I die?' I'd have to be honest with my answer. I'd have to say that people who suffer from Parkinson's tend to live a few years less than people who don't have the disease, but then I'd say they do frequently live to a ripe old age, and most of them live well on into the evening of their years. And that it's not an illness like cancer where you're likely to go within a year or two of diagnosis. It's a slow progressive illness which may give you many years of happy, fulfilled life.

Spinning out time in this way postponed the day of reckoning. Indeed, the many references in doctors' accounts to 'you're likely to die of something else first' indicated that the day of reckoning might be postponed altogether. Several GPs mentioned this, and Dr Naughton's account later showed how he made a joke of it. Initially, however, this was difficult to interpret. I asked Dr Threadgold, who, amidst laughter, said:

> I wish I hadn't said that! I think if someone said that to me I would think wait a minute. That does mean I could die of this. It could get really bad, but what I

actually want to know from this doctor is how likely is it? What's going to happen to me?

The frequent use of this routine suggested that its aim was to reassure (both patient and doctor) and to forestall the distress that dealing with seriously ill P.D. patients undoubtedly evoked. As Dr Fleming noted: 'If he has his heart attack in three years' time and drops dead then I will have felt, well, we've never reached the stage when we had to deal with worse.'

However, other doctors felt more ambivalent. They were aware of the dangers of providing overoptimistic views which subsequent events might render implausible or, as Dr Perlmann noted, involve them in 'the business of telling half lies'. Doctors had to balance possible future challenges to their credibility with the desire to set patients' minds at rest—a task which all doctors thought was part of their caring role. While some doctors disclosed painful and distressing information, no doctor wanted to be gloomy about P.D. to his/her patients. Optimism was therefore qualified. Dr Smythe explained this well:

> Usually, depending on what sort of onset the patient's had, I tend to be more optimistic than pessimistic for them, but I don't give them a very *glowing* picture of saying 'We can get you better, these tablets are going to make you feel great'. The thing I want to draw out of them is not to create a false worry but to allow them to ask about the fears they might have about having the shakes over a long period of time. And then what's going to happen if they get worse.

Doctors here shared the task of managing uncertainty with their patients by giving due weight to the more painful aspects of P.D. in deciding what to explain. The risk of being overoptimistic and being challenged later was much worse than dealing with the anxieties which an open agenda might raise at the time.

Yet this was potentially a tricky issue which involved drawing very fine distinctions. There was less indication that doctors had given the matter the careful consideration that a judgement of this complexity required. Doctors had resolved their doubts and reservations.

Question Responding or Question Initiating?

A further routine in keeping uncertainty in check and thus determining what to communicate was the use of questions. Again doctors in the study varied in their approach. Those doctors with more conservative ideas about communication preferred to respond to patients' questions if and when they occurred. Dr Victor, for example, was confident that 'most of my patients would tell me if they wanted to know something'. Dr Wilkinson said 'I don't say much unless asked', assuming that 'most people actually know about it, I think, or they all seem to'. Dr Dandridge, referring to one of her patients, noted: 'I have not talked to her about it because I think at the moment she has enough on her plate. And I feel that going into too many details wouldn't help at this time. She's intelligent enough to ask if she doesn't know.' Again judgements about patients' levels of intelligence governed how the issue was handled.

Doctors were concerned to protect patients from worrying about 'unnecessary details'. The risk of arousing anxiety—and thus introducing disquiet into the proceedings—was minimized. Dr Naughton felt that sheltering patients from distress was part of his caring role. His account reveals both routines and working beliefs which informed his views about giving explanations—views which, with the candour that characterized our talk, he was prepared to question. He said:

> I would, on the whole, respond to questions as people produce them. I don't tell people things that perhaps they don't want to know and so I don't talk about prognosis with patients, plus the fact that these are usually elderly patients who may well die of something else. If they asked about prognosis I'd be as encouraging and optimistic as possible. I'd say 'Yes, I'm afraid this is a condition that *can* get worse with time', and I usually make a joke and say 'You'll probably get run over by a bus before we need to worry about that'. . . . The more we [Dr Naughton and I] talk, the more I realize I don't say enough.

The onus of widening the field of discussion and allowing a patient's distress to surface was on the patient. However, this process could be circular, as Dr Quinn illustrated:

DR QUINN: I don't believe in telling people when they don't want to know.
R.P.: How do you assess whether they want to know or not?
DR QUINN: When they ask questions.

If patients failed to ask questions, it was assumed that they had none to ask or did not require information. Patients were evidently left to work out the implications of having P.D. for themselves. The device of only responding if a question was asked ensured that difficult decisions about whether or not to broaden the discussion, which might raise uncertainties all round, were unnecessary.

By contrast, other doctors wanted to give patients more room for manoeuvre. They were question initiators, actively concerned to elicit patients' ideas about the illness and to check back on what had been understood in previous discussions or acquired meantime from other sources. Dr Miller's comments were characteristic of GPs following this approach. She had found the exercises currently being developed in medical training particularly helpful:

> I think there are some kinds of 'open sesame' questions that I've found useful, like 'What have you told yourself about this?' or 'What do you think it is?' And certainly in teaching about information, exploring what the other person's ideas are is worth while. You get a completely different conception.

Indeed *not* being alert to patients' signals risked missing vital points in a consultation. She went on:

... what I've found when a patient presents with a headache, at first you can't understand why she's worried. And then you find her husband had a very good friend who was dying with a brain tumour and her headache meant for her that she must have a brain tumour.

She recognized the distinction raised earlier between information-giving as conveying facts and the broader process of facilitating understanding, both for her patients and for herself. It was an important feature of her approach. In order to encourage patients' understanding, she needed pointers from patients to guide her. But she was ready to respond to them openly. Such a shared approach to understanding reduced any anxiety to which the use of open questions might otherwise expose doctors.

COMMENT

Routines thus helped to soften the impact of conveying sensitive information to patients. Their use enabled those GPs who preferred a closed approach to avoid being explicit about the prognosis. Those with a more open approach managed uncertainty by meeting patients half-way.

SUMMARY AND COMMENT

The evidence shows that uncertainty and its management was important in determining what doctors thought they should explain to patients about the implications of having P.D. However, although doctors were faced with uncertain choices, this does not imply that they were consumed with indecision in thinking about their work. In their accounts doctors showed that they had developed ways of imposing order on potential disorder. However, uncertainty was managed differently by the doctors in the study, indicating very different policies on communicating information.

For those doctors who wanted to keep discussion within acceptable limits, the use of broad judgements and routines and appeals to the 'obviousness' of experience helped to reduce ambiguity and simplified explanation-giving. The development of a 'house style' to suit all-comers absolved them from having to make difficult and potentially anxiety-laden decisions in individual cases. Indeed, its very use was at variance with the notion of treating patients as individuals. Explanations either were seen as unnecessary or were given in very simple, general terms (see Taylor, 1988). Doctors wanted to shield their patients from the impact of possibly distressing information. In doing so they protected themselves from the anxiety of handling an unknown—and perhaps feared—response. Age, intelligence, the use of optimism and question-responding rather than question initiation figured prominently in these GPs' policies. Stereotypes about age were plainly taken for granted. Not only was disability seen to be comparatively less distressing for the elderly; one disability, as it were, cancelled out the other. This had important consequences: older people were not always seen to require as much communication as younger patients.

Some doctors had a middle-of-the-road approach. They often acknowledged the complexity of explanation-giving but had resolved anxieties, usually in favour of containing the flow of information to patients, so that they could cope.

Other doctors had more flexible policies. Their ideas about patients were more open to question—sometimes uncomfortably so. Indeed some assumptions were turned on their head. A counselling-oriented approach seemed to enable doctors to handle the inevitable distress to patients of disclosing painful information—a point I shall explore in further detail in Chapter 6.

These GPs felt that patients could cope with explanations, provided they were sensitively tailored to a patient's changing needs. Patients were regarded as competent adults, capable, with help, of handling distressing information. There was a presumption of openness. Doctors felt that open explanations which acknowledged distress helped patients to cope better in the long run. Frankness reduced anxieties on the part of doctors too. They were not placed in difficult positions of remembering who had been told what. Further, by widening the discussion, doctors could learn from patients what was troubling them and thus target their explanations more effectively. Openness enabled both patient and doctor to cope better. The management of uncertainty was a task to be shared between patient and doctor, helping to defuse the situation all round.

An important issue was highlighted by Dr Quinn. It concerned the difference, not always appreciated, between knowledge and understanding—between the process of conveying information as a series of discrete facts and that of enabling patients to understand what those facts meant in terms of their own lives. Doctors needed to facilitate this translation process. To do this well requires an understanding of the patient as a person. As we have seen, this was not always forthcoming.

However, any professional must minimize his/her decision-making problems. The question was to what extent doctors' management of uncertainty was likely to enhance or hinder the ability to respond to patients' needs. While understanding the wishes of those with more closed policies to protect patients from distress, my argument is that those with more flexible policies were more likely to be able to respond appropriately—to cater both for those who wanted to know and for those who did not. How well doctors' views about what to tell corresponded with what patients said they wanted will emerge in the following chapter.

3
Understanding the Implications: Knowledge as a Resource?

INTRODUCTION

At one stage in our talks Mrs Jenson said:

> No way could I find anybody anywhere that could give the relatives information on what to expect. Does it go through stages, or does it just gradually go downhill? . . . As it stands at the moment there is nobody, but nobody that I can talk to on any level anywhere. It's taken me so much time to get it clear in my mind.

On the face of it, her *cri de coeur* required a simple, direct response: the provision of information. Yet, as we shall see, the situation was not nearly so straightforward.

The previous chapter has shown how GPs reduced the potential ambiguity and discomfort of giving explanations by the use of beliefs and routines. For patients, the experience and management of the uncertainties involved in understanding what to expect were crucially different.

With the diagnosis of his/her illness, the patient faces new uncertainties. What is likely to happen, and when? What does it mean for everyday life, work and the family? What about the future? What help can be expected from the patient's GP in resolving these questions?

One way of reducing anxiety is by obtaining information. Studies on chronic illness amply attest to the value of knowledge as a resource (Power and Sax, 1978; Schneider and Conrad, 1983; Jobling and Coles, 1988; Robinson, 1988). As we shall see, the situation was much more complex. Coming to terms with what the facts mean is a subtle process which, I believe, has been partly obscured behind broad, oversimplified demands for more open information exchange between patient and doctor. Knowledge could be a mixed blessing.

This chapter explores the various strategies patients in the study adopted to deal with the uncertainties of what to expect. It addresses the following questions: How much did patients want to know, in what detail and at what stage in their illness? When did patients not want to know, and how did they manage information they were not ready to assimilate? I then examine the extent to which patients saw their GPs as being alert and sensitive to their information needs.

For the purposes of analysis, responses fell into three groups:

(1) Seekers: those patients who actively sought to discover what was likely to happen. The task often involved sustained research from medical and lay sources. The certainty of something bad was preferable to the uncertainty of not knowing.

(2) Weavers: those patients whose needs for information fluctuated. Sometimes they felt able to assimilate additional facts about P.D.; at other times they preferred not to know. Information was selectively interpreted to allow patients to turn knowledge to their own advantage.

(3) Avoiders: those patients who deliberately chose not to find out the implications. The anxiety of not knowing was preferable to the risk of having their private, often unacknowledged, fears about the illness confirmed.

However, these must not be seen as fixed, discrete categories. Patients varied in their responses over time, sometimes wanting to know 'the truth', at other times settling for a version of reality which was sufficient to allay anxiety and retain hope, and sometimes rejecting the facts altogether. However, these were the main strategies to emerge.

INFORMATION: FRIEND OR FOE?

Seekers: *'If the patient knows what's happening and is going to happen they can help themselves adjust better to cope with the disease'*

Five patients in the study could be described as Seekers, or to have had a period of Seekership in that they tried to manage uncertainty by a deliberate search for information. Their anxiety was so overwhelming that they could not contain the urgency of finding out what to expect. The newly acquired label, 'Parkinson's patient', could not be incorporated into their identity without a clear knowledge of the implications of the illness.

Mr Grenville described how it affected him:

My determination and drive were so great to get to know as much about the disease as possible that I went to the University Library and got out books containing papers, past references on Parkinson's, of which I must have understood about twenty per cent, but the drive sustained me. . . . Immediately I accepted that something was wrong I was engaged in rigorous research for my own understanding and journey of discovery to find out what its nature was.

It was *re*search as much as a search which preoccupied him (Darling, 1979). The value of information as a means of gaining a purchase on what was happening was pivotal. Initially research provided a vantage point from which strategies to manage the implications of the illness (and ultimately the uncertainties and distress of the illness experience itself) could be evolved. However, Mr Grenville commented 'it was only over time that the background got filled in'. Eight years after his diagnosis, there were still some unanswered questions.

Even with personal experience of the illness, Mr Canning discovered that the search for information often raised as many questions as it answered. He said: 'I learnt the lot on my own. I thought I knew more than the average person because of my mother [who had Parkinson's], but when I started reading I learned with horror that I didn't know anything about it at all.' Each new door opened up further uncertainties. Moreover, there was a gulf between what Mr Canning knew from personal experience and the apparently conflicting and imprecise information, particularly concerning the treatment, which he discovered on reading. Medical uncertainty added a new dimension to what patients thought was merely ignorance on their part. The situation was not improved for him at the time of diagnosis, where he felt he had been misled by false optimism:

> The thing was that he [consultant] built me up into this euphoric state by saying it was mild and then when I got home I realized it was a let-down. . . . Your immediate reaction is that you've got mild P.D. and it might stay the same for the next twenty years, and then you start reading deeper into it and you realize that everyone has mild Parkinson's, to start with anyway.

For Seekers, these discoveries often led to intense frustration, affecting all areas of a patient's life. Mr Canning had been obliged to abandon his treasured plans for retirement. However, when active strategies to resolve uncertainty simply raised new doubts, patients were thrown back on their own resources to try and understand what was happening. Anxiety was heightened.

Mrs Pembridge felt similarly driven to find out the implications of the label, only to discover that she had taken on more than she had bargained for. P.D., being generally less well known, does not necessarily inspire such immediate dread and terror as does cancer, for instance. Mrs Pembridge was not prepared for the devastating image which confronted her. She described her search for information:

MRS PEMBRIDGE: I was so shattered when I came out of the clinic I went straight into a bookshop to find out what it was all about. And one of the things I read was that your handwriting becomes very small. Mine was so small that I could hardly read it. I read all about these different things. I felt even more shattered.
R.P.: With hindsight, do you feel it was a good idea to go and read about it straight away? Some people do it other ways.

MRS PEMBRIDGE: I had to. I had to find out for myself, didn't I. I wanted to know the major symptoms. If I hadn't found out I would have been so mystified. . . . I'm not sorry I found out that way. Because I hadn't got the symptoms I thought I'm not that bad.

Knowledge proved to be a mixed blessing. While it settled anxiety on one score (she now knew the worst that could happen), it raised anxiety on others: how would she cope? Her last remark, however, was significant. She had chiselled hope out of a seemingly forlorn situation by contrasting her own physical condition with that described in the books she found. As she was comparatively mildly handicapped at that stage, she felt this was a perfectly reasonable interpretation to make. The picture was not entirely bleak. She was thus able to distance herself from the enormity of absorbing all the facts at once.

COMMENT

With diagnosis, biographical wholeness had been shattered. Some patients could not form a coherent picture of themselves until uncertainties had been clarified. For them knowledge was a vital means of dealing with anxiety. It helped patients to establish a measure of control over what was happening.

However, Seekership had its problems. It brought patients face to face with medical uncertainty, often leaving them feeling frustrated and help-less. Some patients were exasperated by the lack of certainty in the prognosis. However, others found that their quest for certainty had gone too far. The truth was too brutal. In this sense, Seekers had much in common with Weavers.

Weavers: *'Progression is something you know but you don't know, if you see what I mean'*

Six patients and their spouses managed uncertainty by trying to control the pace with which information was acquired rather differently. They edged their way forward, selecting pieces of information which they could absorb, sometimes settling for a truth which was less than the whole truth, until they felt ready to move on again. It was a precarious position to maintain. Events occurred which struck a discordant note. Often patients were confronted willy-nilly with images of 'this could be me in five years' time', forcing an awareness that was premature.

The oscillating nature of both wanting and not wanting to know was well illustrated by Mrs Franklin:

I was only able to absorb so much at the beginning. You take so much of it in, then you get over that, then you take a bit more in and so on. Then you get to a stage where you think you've heard and seen the worst. Then I found I could really get down to it and read about it, and perhaps start to climb back again, which is what happened.

When she developed muscle cramps, the desire to resolve the mystery overcame the fear of what she might discover in the process. She found to her pleasure that reading restored her confidence. The information gained also equipped her with a vocabulary to discuss her problems with her consultant 'in accurate terms'. She was no longer groping in the dark. Knowledge was ultimately richly rewarding in reducing her anxiety and helping her gain a purchase over what was happening.

Mr and Mrs Mitchell, however, had had a more trying time. They described the difficulties they had found in asking questions about a condition of which they knew little. Our talks were punctuated by the refrain 'We don't know what to expect'. Anxiety was such that I gave them Godwin-Austen's (1984) book to read. Evidently resolving the uncertainty to a degree had been helpful. Mr Mitchell thought:

> It's helped me in such a way that I can understand better now which I didn't before. And all the symptoms that I had I now realize what caused them. . . . It's not a killer disease which I thought it was in the first place. I thought it was a wasting disease, you wasted away and you sort of died. But it's not like that. . . .
> The future, it looks a lot brighter for me in that respect with Parkinson's, through understanding more. I understand it more so that I can cope with it. Cope with what comes along. You must know about it to cope with it.

Both Mr and Mrs Mitchell said they felt reassured by what they had read. However, it was apparent that this was quite sufficient for the time being. It had answered questions Mr Mitchell had been unable to formulate and articulate, but was evidently still sufficiently general for him to interpret the information to his advantage.

The timing of information discovery was crucial. It was apparent that Mrs Jenson had not always been as unequivocal about finding out what to expect as her opening remark might suggest. The drive for information was only triggered by a crisis following Mr Jenson's bowel operation, when she said: '*Now* we would like to know. Now I would because I'm over the hump. The worst thing is not knowing which to blame for what. It would be easy to attribute everything to Parkinson's. But I don't know which is which. The doctors won't say. He's just weak.'

The added burden of a new set of circumstances aroused greater anxiety and prompted more determined efforts by Mrs Jenson to 'get to the bottom of it'. Until his death she accompanied her husband to hospital appointments to ask questions, and was determined not to be 'side-tracked with vague generalizations'. Prevarication no longer allayed her rising anxieties.

Patients also equivocated over the amount of information they could cope with at any one time. While some wanted broad indications of the outlook, they did not necessarily want explicit details. For instance, Mrs Quentin said: 'You want information to go in but you don't want it hammered in.' Mrs Unwin echoed this feeling: 'You don't want your nose rubbed in it, do you?'

Sometimes patients knew—as Mr Unwin knew from personal experience of his brother-in-law, who was seriously handicapped with P.D.—but saw themselves as different. Elaborate distancing strategies allowed Mr and Mrs Unwin to separate the two strands of experience, even though Mr Unwin was wheelchair-bound for much of the day and his speech was often barely comprehensible.

MRS UNWIN: It varies so much, doesn't it. It doesn't affect everyone the same, you know. He knew he wouldn't be like his brother-in-law.
MR UNWIN: You think you're going to be lucky. It might not get too bad.
MRS UNWIN: It doesn't mean it's going to happen to you anyway. It might happen to some. It might not happen to you.

They managed uncertainty by selecting pieces of information which fitted their interpretation of the situation at any given time (see Roth, 1963; McIntosh, 1977). The variability of their prognosis allowed for such reasoning. Each case was unique. At the same time, regardless of the degree of physical impairment, patients could carry on so long as they did not dwell on the possibility of their condition deteriorating any further.

It might be tempting to attribute a note of desperation to their remarks. Indeed, apparent denial of the physical reality of their condition calls into question the very nature of rationality. How was it that patients could hold images of themselves which were at variance with how others might see them? I believe that such a simple reading of their comments underestimates the necessity for, and tenacity of, people's survival strategies. As Wiener (1975) and Robinson (1988) have noted of their patients with rheumatoid arthritis and multiple sclerosis, respectively, 'denial' was less a dismissal of the condition itself than of its personal and social significance. Patients assessed what might happen to their bodies in ways which enabled them to hold on to a sense of who they were. It was a perfectly rational approach, consistent with their attempt to minimize anxiety and preserve hope.

The problem of handling information which was at odds with how patients chose to see themselves affected both Weavers and Avoiders. Both positions were precarious. It was not always possible to avoid visits to out-patient clinics, where patients were confronted with others in a more parlous state than themselves. Mr Dempsey, for instance, had developed quite elaborate 'switching-off' tactics over the years. He described his visits to the hospital clinic:

I get a bit worried when I go up to the hospital and see other people much further advanced and I think to myself and wonder because these people tell me they was just like me a few years previous, and I think to myself 'Oh blimey!' I just sort of close my mind down on it and think about something else and hope for the best. You must have a mechanism that you switch off.

A more extreme situation had arisen for Mr Jenson. Some two years after his diagnosis, he was taken on a tour of a hospital ward for P.D. patients, where he was '. . . thrown in at the deep end amongst all the sufferers in various stages of development of the disease . . . rubbing shoulders with people suffering in a much more serious way, wheelchairs, lack of speech control . . .'. Apparently, little had been explained and the experience had left him bewildered and confused. However, he had comforted himself with the thought that his own condition bore little resemblance to that of the patients seen. Reference to his own comparative lack of handicap at the time bolstered this notion. He was able to say 'Of course I didn't realize all the implications at the time'.

Patients were thus engaged in separating what they felt were quite different strands of experience. Being able to say not only 'this is not me' but also 'this is not going to be me' allowed them to manage the fears such experiences undoubtedly aroused.

COMMENT

Weavers were engaged in a precarious balancing act: between allowing in sufficient information to alleviate uncertainty and ensuring that there was enough leeway to maintain hope. The timing of discovery was thus crucial in determining whether information was helpful or harmful. Some information aggravated anxiety and patients adopted ways of disregarding experiences at variance with how they chose to see themselves. At other times a crisis prompted a search for more information, involving Weavers in strategies more akin to those of Seekers. Knowledge was often only seen retrospectively as a useful resource.

It would be misleading to describe such manoeuvres pejoratively as an unhealthy, if not pathological, denial to be worked through. For these patients they formed a vital part of their survival kit—and in this they had much in common with Avoiders.

Avoiders: *'I think probably I'd have been more unhappy. There was a long period when I was being treated. I mean I was happy, however you choose to define happiness'*

Three patients, and the wife of one patient, chose not to know the implications of having P.D. This came as a surprise, as it challenged my own views about the right to know—even a moral imperative that one ought to know—if not for oneself, then for the sake of family and friends. Knowledge, however, was not seen as a means of alleviating anxiety. It was a potential threat to these patients. They preferred the uncertainty of not knowing, because it was this uncertainty which gave them hope (see McIntosh, 1977). Yet, as with those pursuing Seekership or Weaving strategies, fear was often lurking near the surface.

Mr Irving and Mr Richards only modified their position when physical deterioration made it impossible to ignore the implications any longer. Initially, however, Avoiding worked well for patients who were still relatively unimpaired. Mr Irving reflected:

> Looking back on it I was very incurious about what the long-term effects were. I just thought 'Well, I've got an illness and the pills seem to be working and I'll just put up with that'. . . . I thought whatever's wrong is being put right. There was no need to bother about it unduly. Get on with what I was doing.

He managed uncertainty by ignoring the significance of the condition for his everyday life, a position helped by early successful treatment. He had not wanted to question his consultant, and appreciated the latter's concentration on 'making sure I got the right treatment'. He did not regret the decision in retrospect. It was only when he 'got stuck' for the first time that he realized 'I wasn't going back to the stage where it was never going to happen again'. Only then did he seek information to try and grasp what was happening.

Mr and Mrs Richards made a more active decision not to know. Mrs Richards explained:

> Well, I had the feeling that the future could be rather bad for my husband, but since it was a mild case. . . . A friend of a relative had Parkinson's and we heard things about him which didn't make us very happy. So we didn't want to delve into things and let it cloud our minds and make us unhappy now. I just want us to make the best of this period when things are working reasonably well not to cloud our minds with all the possibilities that could come up. If it's to be in the future let it *be* in the future. . . . As I understand it Parkinson's is not just a disease which is all cut and dried. There are facets and people can be slightly this and slightly that. As his thyroid specialist said to him 'I understand you're a Parkinsonian'. He hasn't got Parkinson's *Disease*, but you're a Parkinsonian which is slightly different.

Patients would rather be unaware of the implications, however much anxiety this might cause, than risk facing information which might overwhelm them. They postponed facing reality by viewing their own case as different, relying here on a distinction between 'having the Disease' and 'being a Parkinsonian'. Why meet trouble half-way? The couple selected favourable cues from what they were obliged to hear to allay anxiety for the time being. The future was put into cold storage.

Interestingly, Mr and Mrs Richards's position changed over the months I saw them. Mrs Richards suddenly asked what the side-effects of the treatment were. The constantly evolving nature of what seemed initially to be quite stable information needs cannot be sufficiently stressed.

After her husband's death, Mrs Richards reflected on the wisdom of their policy. The possibility that information might have been helpful bothered her, but on balance it seemed that the happiness they shared until shortly before his death more than compensated for the lack of help. The memory of her happy times nursing her husband sustained Mrs Richards in her grief.

However, fear was never far from the surface. While Mrs Richards claimed 'I went along with it simply through fear, because I was afraid to know', fear had left Mrs York almost paralysed. She had been unable to question either her GP or her consultant—a policy which accorded well with her husband's sanguine views on life. She made no further efforts to find out about the implications: 'I was too frightened. I'm too frightened to ask very much about anything. I'd just as soon in life go along and let it happen. I don't want to anticipate any more horrors that I've got to cope with'. These fears in time were well justified, as her husband deteriorated rapidly. A year after our talks he was in a nursing home.

Despite what Mr Dempsey knew from the experience of his mother's and grandmother's P.D., he placed a quite definite embargo on all further information—unless, and until, his condition worsened. After twelve years with the illness, he was still comparatively well and looking after himself. The prospect of having to assimilate any further information was profoundly threatening:

> I certainly wouldn't like someone to tell me all the things that could go wrong with this Parkinson's because I'd worry myself sick about it. If I get it I get it, and if I don't—twelve years have gone by and I'm still mobile and like I said I've still got my noodle. I'd rather carry on living the way I am, perhaps kidding myself. Live for today and worry about tomorrow tomorrow.

The passage of time had not caused the deterioration he had feared initially. Armed with this knowledge, he could discount the experiences of his less fortunate colleagues. He had outwitted the future.

COMMENT

Avoiders managed uncertainty by choosing not to know. They preferred to remain in the dark rather than risk the possibility of facing a prognosis which might destroy all hope. Knowledge, far from being a resource, was a positive threat, and patients devised elaborate strategies to handle any information which might jeopardize their position. In retrospect, the period of not knowing was not generally regretted. It gave patients and their relatives a vital breathing space in which to live as normally as possible. The right not to know was as important as the right to know.

Thus, the idea of a neat linear progression from a state of ignorance, through gradual awareness to a full, 'mature' acceptance of having P.D.

hardly accords with the complex feelings of the patients described in the study. Patients wove in and out of phases over time, sometimes even unlearning information in an effort to impose order on their experience.

THE ROLE OF THE GP

The crucial question is: How far did patients in the study feel their own GPs supported their struggles to handle the uncertainties and anxieties in discovering what to expect? Evaluations were complex. They were, of course, partly a product of patients' previous experiences. The situation was also complicated by the presence or absence of a consultant in managing their P.D. Patients considered themselves variously as 'being under the hospital', 'being under the hospital and the doctor' or 'being under the GP'.

It has often been assumed that patients are unable, or do not want, to assess the technical competence of their GPs, and that GPs are valued primarily for their affective skills. Several studies, however, have documented patients' lack of confidence in their GPs' ability to treat less ordinary complaints (see, for example, Comaroff and Maguire's 1981 study of parents of children with leukaemia, and Speedling's 1982 study of heart attack patients). Others have shown how patients have found themselves teaching their GPs about the details of their particular condition (Schneider and Conrad, 1983; Kelly, 1987; Oliver *et al.*, 1988).

I shall show that patients in the study evaluated both technical and affective skills. Moreover, the presence or absence of clinical experience in handling P.D. had important consequences for future relationships. They often determined whether GPs were approached for help with deeper, personal problems raised by the illness. There were two broad responses. Patients either saw their GP as inexperienced in handling such a complex illness (two thirds of those in the study) or, by contrast, were confident in their GP's expertise and valued his support.

A lack of experience: *'I just don't think they understand. But they don't* know *they don't understand!'*

Nine patients saw their GPs as unfamiliar with P.D. Sometimes this realization occurred at the outset. Mr Dempsey, for instance, approached his GP with fairly clear ideas of what was wrong. He was immediately referred to a neurologist, a decision he was pleased with: 'After him telling me he wasn't really skilled in it, I didn't really think he was the best person to handle it. It's like calling a plumber and then the plumber sending a cowboy in to do the job, isn't it.' He regarded the relation between GP and consultant as one of 'apprentice and a skilled man'.

Other patients had had little confidence in their GP to start with. Mr Grenville commented:

> I think I somehow never expected the GP to know anything about it. Possibly because the doctor friend had already tuned me in to seeing a specialist. . . . But the GP readily admitted to not knowing what it was. . . . I've had experience of GPs in the realm of schizophrenia. That encouraged me to form the impression that if Parkinson's is in a similar category one shouldn't expect doctors to be competent beyond offering prescriptions according to guidance from the consultant.

Patients did not consider a GP to be appropriate to handle such a complex illness. Similarly, Mr Vernon, although liking and respecting his GP, did not often consult him about P.D. While he felt his GP had become more familiar with the technicalities of the illness over time, he thought it impossible for any GP to appreciate 'all the finer twists and twiddles that may only work in certain circumstances'. With such views, the framework in which a meaningful dialogue between patient and doctor could take place was absent.

These patients often found that their GPs' inexperience was more apparent as the illness unfolded and they themselves became better informed. Mr Canning, after a week's anxious deliberations, had changed his GP a year after the onset of P.D. He thought his present GP was honest about his unfamiliarity with the illness, but was prepared to remedy this. They had struck up a partnership. As a result, Mr Canning's frustration at the inexperience of his previous GP was somewhat mollified:

> My GP doesn't know what he's doing, but it's nice to know he doesn't and that he'll read the same book as I will and we can discuss it as intelligent people. I quoted something and I got the figures wrong and so he immediately grabbed the book, started looking it up and I said 'Well, it's page 177'. He knew that I could really be regarded as equal. So now he doesn't even pretend he knows.

The idea of the patient–doctor relationship being a partnership where both parties worked together in managing the delicate task of discovery appealed to patients. It enhanced trust rather than otherwise, and helped to compensate patients for the shock of realising that their GPs were sometimes unfamiliar with the condition.

However, where little or no interest was seen to be shown, unfamiliarity with P.D. had distressing effects. Mrs Pembridge, for instance, desperate for reassurance, had approached her GP early on to supplement the information she had gleaned from reading books in W. H. Smith's. She recalled asking:

> Mrs Pembridge: I said 'Can you tell me something about this illness?' He said 'It's very complicated'. He got this book down from the shelf but then he told me nothing. . . . I assumed he didn't know anything about it. He said 'I'm not a neurologist'. The times he's said that to me! Whenever I ask him questions he says 'Ask the neurologist'.

R.P.: What does that make you feel?
Mrs Pembridge: He doesn't want to know. Don't ask me why. I just feel that.

When she discovered that her GP seemed unwilling to try, she was profoundly distressed. Apparent lack of interest was equated with lack of care and concern. It had long-term consequences. Mrs Pembridge had avoided contact with her GP for several years since diagnosis. When I talked with her a year later, however, her attitude had changed. With her move to sheltered accommodation, she found her GP beginning to take an interest. 'He must have been feeling guilty', she mused. The seriousness of her complaint had been appreciated for the first time: she was 'really ill'. She was upset that it had not been so, perhaps when she most needed it.

Two patients recalled particular incidents which had forced them to recognize their respective GPs' inexperience. Mr Irving, for instance, had considered his GP 'affable enough' until he 'got stuck' on the surgery stairs on one occasion and found he needed help: 'He obviously hadn't seen anyone in a frozen position before. And it was quite a surprise to him that I couldn't move at all'. If GPs were seen as inexperienced, patients felt bereft as far as any sensitive response to their information needs was concerned. Moreover, when patients lost confidence in their GPs' clinical competence and ability to explain what was happening, they also saw their GPs as inappropriate to help in other aspects of the illness where, ideally, doctors might have come into their own. Mr Irving summed up his thoughts: 'He'd not be my first port of call. My GP was less helpful than I thought when I first ticked your card [Chapter 9]. It's my fault because I never bother him with it because he doesn't know much. If I felt he knew more then I'd be encouraged.' Again patients' assessments of their GPs changed over time. A single response did not do justice to what patients felt as the illness progressed.

The system in which patients found themselves also increased uncertainty and hampered the development of a patient–doctor relationship where anxiety about the implications of having P.D. might have been sensitively handled. Four patients felt they were 'under the hospital'. Even though Mr Richards, for example, wanted to talk with his GP—he was evidently ambivalent about Avoiding—he thought information from the hospital would 'get lost in the system', leaving his GP unaware of the latest developments, particularly in his medication.

Lack of liaison was also seen as an excuse on the part of Mr and Mrs Mitchell's GP not to get involved. It demonstrated a clear lack of interest and concern:

Mr Mitchell: I thought my own GP would help in explaining to you and give me more help with the tablets. All he says though is that he'll leave the hospital to deal with the tablets and all.

MRS MITCHELL: He's wondering where he stands. Instead of the doctor being helpful, he's not.
MR MITCHELL: The thing is if you go and ask him what it is he won't tell you nothing at all because he reckons he hasn't got notes or letters from the hospital.
MRS MITCHELL: The hospital writes to him, but for some unknown reason he don't receive them, if you can believe it.

Not only was 'the system' anxiety-provoking for patients. Some GPs' responses within the system discouraged patients from turning to their GPs for help in coming to terms with the implications of having P.D.

Thus, the perceived inappropriateness of these patients' GPs to deal with a condition of this complexity, unfamiliarity with the illness (well acknowledged in the profession: Thompson, 1987; and attested to by some patients: Essex, 1983) and difficulties in 'the system' meant that patients who sought help from their GPs had to go elsewhere. This had serious consequences for future patient–GP communication, particularly for Seekers and Weavers. Not only was the framework in which to respond sensitively to patients' information needs absent; patients did not feel inclined to seek help with deeper personal problems which the illness raised—an area where GPs were uniquely placed to help. For these patients, uncertainty at best had not been addressed; at worst it had been heightened.

Support and Reassurance: *'He's always there in the background if you want him'*

By contrast, the presence of a caring, supportive GP who was sensitive to the anxieties which too much or too little information might cause made a crucial difference to four other patients' ability to handle the uncertainties of discovery.

Support in this sensitive area often involved quite intangible aspects of human relationships, such as a GP's availability, and his/her willingness to give time and to demonstrate interest, care and concern. These patients felt that their GPs understood the distress a knowledge of what to expect could cause, enabling Seekers to obtain speedy information, helping Weavers assimilate information when they were ready to do so and protecting Avoiders from being overwhelmed with information they did not want. Basic competence was not in doubt. Moreover, patients were not obliged to wait often lengthy intervals for hospital appointments before they could discuss their anxieties. The GP was accessible to provide continuing support. Miss Evans thought:

I've had things explained to me as I've developed the symptoms. My GP understands it very well. He knows what I'm talking about. I feel he understands perfectly how I feel. I get the impression that he knows quite a lot about it. He's not an old doctor. He's probably more up-to-date than others. I don't feel worried when I go into the surgery that he's going to be off-hand. I know that he'll do what he can to help.

This understanding supplemented her own professional knowledge as a nurse and proceeded, step by step, in encouraging new understanding as the illness unfolded. The demonstration of care—never feeling rebuffed—combined with trust in his basic competence paved the way for a continuing, supportive relationship.

Mrs Quentin particularly appreciated her GP's efforts to explain what to expect, after her consultant had passed the onus of telling the diagnosis back to her GP:

He was so kind and he talked to me about it. He knows as much as any GP about the Disease. He doesn't know what causes the symptoms, of course, but he asks you, he does question you. I like it because he's never afraid to get a book out in front of one. I think that's good. He never seems to be in a hurry to get rid of you.

When patients' GPs admitted their own personal uncertainty and indicated that they were willing to look things up, this enhanced rather than reduced patients' confidence. It showed that doctors had a human face and cared sufficiently for their patients to try and familiarize themselves with conditions about which they were unsure.

Mr and Mrs Unwin were similarly pleased with their GP's explanations, which both complemented and enabled them to distance themselves from their personal experience of Mr Unwin's brother-in-law. Their GP evidently understood their fears of being overwhelmed with too much information:

Mrs Unwin: I think there's a lot he doesn't say you wouldn't like to hear really.
R.P.: You think there are some things best left unsaid?
Mr and Mrs Unwin (*in unison*): Mmmmm.
Mrs Unwin: There's a lot of psychology to Dr X. He notices everything.

These patients saw their GPs as alert and sensitive to the anxieties that understanding information might arouse. The ability of GPs to work at patients' own time and pace, and knowing where to stop and wait, were crucial in providing a framework where anxieties could be contained. As a result, patients had rich and lasting relationships with their GPs.

SUMMARY AND COMMENT

This chapter has considered how patients handled the uncertainty of finding out what the implications of the illness were, and how far they felt their own GPs helped in the process. The timing, extent and explicitness of coming to understand what the facts meant had to be managed. Patients evolved strategies which tended to reflect both a general outlook on life and a specific response to the demands of this situation. These were crucial in enabling patients to impose order on disorder.

Contrary to much of the literature, information was not uniformly seen as a resource in alleviating anxiety. Patients' accounts eloquently showed how their thoughts changed over time, sometimes expanding, sometimes modifying what they were able to take on. The process was far from linear in the sense of patients progressing neatly from a state of ignorance to one of full awareness. Nor was it complete. Awareness was often partial, and patients sometimes unlearnt information, reversing positions.

Nevertheless, broad patterns were identified. Seekers could not come to terms with the illness without information, and saw its acquisition as a means of achieving this. They often felt frustrated by the imprecision of the facts that were available. Weavers tried to pace the process of assimilating information as they went along, striking hazardous balances between maintaining hope and alleviating uncertainty. Patients developed quite elaborate strategies to disregard information which contradicted how they chose to see themselves. Avoiders kept anxiety at bay by postponing the day of reckoning as long as possible. They preferred not to know what to expect rather than risk being confronted with a possibly distressing prognosis. Knowledge, far from being important in reducing anxiety, heightened it.

GPs who were sensitively attuned to what was happening played a vital role in helping four patients manage the anxieties in understanding the implications of the illness. Both affective skills and technical competence were necessary for the GP to be seen as helpful. Warmth, care and understanding on their own were insufficient. Patients needed to feel that the GP knew what he was doing. Otherwise the sensitive task of responding to a patient's needs could not even start. It is not just a GP's niceness that is at stake.

Where clinical experience, or the willingness to acquire it, were absent, patients went elsewhere. Thus, unfamiliarity with the illness, together with difficulties in 'the system', could have disturbing consequences for any future patient–GP relationship. Patients were unlikely to turn to their GP for any further help.

Lack of familiarity with the condition may be relatively easy to remedy. The intangibles of communication between patient and doctor may be less amenable to change. Both the developing pattern of patients' needs and the complexity of their responses indicated that the task of conveying information had to be handled with the utmost delicacy. Where GPs were unable to address such needs, patients were often profoundly distressed.

This evidence raises the broader policy question of how far patients can be responded to as individuals in a system of general practice which is becoming increasingly bureaucratized. As the previous chapter indicated, the beliefs and routines used, particularly by doctors with a more closed approach, suggested that they were not. The responses of doctors who were more flexible, on the other hand, indicated they could be: the potential was there. As I show in the following chapters, the emergence of the patient-as-person is vitally important to an understanding of a satisfactory patient–GP relationship.

4
The Drug Regimen: 'We Can Treat It'

INTRODUCTION

The problems of deciding what to tell patients about the implications of P.D. which were explored in Chapter 2 were compounded by the further difficulties of deciding what to explain and how to supervise the drug treatment. We have seen in Chapter 1 that, technically, management of the drug regimen is complex, requiring fine tuning over time to achieve the best balance between minimizing the side-effects and maximizing control of the illness. Clinically this demands careful individual assessment.

The side-effects of the drugs, the difficulty in accurately predicting their effects in any one individual and their decreasing efficacy over time also raised potentially much more difficult questions for doctors: what to tell patients about the drugs; how to weigh up the perceived costs and benefits over the short, medium and longer term; and how to mediate between patient and doctor claims to expertise in the daily management of the treatment. GPs did not know how their patients were going to react, either physically or psychologically. The situation faced by the GP was potentially highly unpredictable.

This chapter explores first the way explanations about the rationale and the side-effects of the medication were best seen to be conveyed. Second, it examines GPs' ideas about how far patients should be encouraged to take responsibility for the daily management of their treatment. As before, I shall focus on the beliefs held and routines GPs developed to deal with potential uncertainty and anxiety, and their implications for communication.

RATIONALE AND SIDE-EFFECTS

The Rationale: *'Anyone in my experience is glad to take them'*

Thirteen GPs in the study claimed that they gave a general justification for using the treatment to their patients. However, doctors' policies again

41

varied. Some felt that the medication could best be managed by disclosing little information about the drugs—a pattern found in treatment of conditions such as epilepsy (Schneider and Conrad, 1983), rheumatoid arthritis (Locker, 1983) and hypertension (Zola, 1983). Consistent with their policies about explaining what to expect of the illness, Dr Dandridge and Dr Victor felt that patients should be protected from the impact of distressing information. They based their judgements on what they thought was in their patients' best interests. Dr Victor, referring to one of his patients handicapped with both arthritis and P.D., recalled:

> I said 'Well I can give you something, never mind the arthritis, I think that might make you walk a bit better'. So I put him on some Sinemet and said 'Come and see me in a month' and he said 'Oh, I feel much better. I'm walking better than I've done for ages.'

When asked whether he had explained anything about Sinemet, Dr Victor continued: 'I'm not sure that there's much point in telling them.' He assumed that patients preferred not to know and that things were better handled that way. A caring role was a protective one. Non-disclosure of anxiety-provoking information also ensured that any uncertainty was kept at bay. The evident effectiveness of this approach was justified by the very tangible feedback Dr Victor received.

However, other doctors considered that providing a very broad outline was useful, particularly in ensuring compliance where patients might be reluctant to take pills for life. Dr Ogilvie thought that such an approach might best be put across this way:

> I'd want to explain what the drugs were and how they are a recent innovation and that they have transformed the lives of many Parkinson's sufferers, and that they can make a lot of difference although they're not a cure. But they can help a great deal. I would explain my reasons for giving them—that the disease is interfering with their life-style, in other words that it was important that we should seek to try and prevent that and that these tablets, whilst not a cure, could help in that situation.

The package was presented to patients so as to ensure their co-operation. It was in the patient's interests to take the treatment. He believed that its benefits outweighed any possible costs. However, this was not a calculation he felt was appropriate to discuss with patients. It would have raised difficult issues, the outcome of which might have been less amenable to control. The difficulties of the medication were played down. Again doctors wanted to shield their patients from distress.

At the same time, these doctors were concerned to alert their patients, in non-specific ways, to the possibility of differences in response, thereby introducing an *element* of uncertainty into patients' ideas about the efficacy of treatment, while simultaneously indicating that everything was under control. Dr Fleming said, for instance:

I do at some point say to patients that in giving you this drug there's a certain amount of trial and error. And you've got to make it clear that by that you don't mean it's experimentation. Patients don't like to feel they're being experimented on. But there is a certain amount of trial and error. You may respond to treatment, you may not. What I tend to say is that I don't think this drug in the dose I've given you will upset you. If it does upset you it may be this way or that, and if that happens then come back to me and tell me what's happening.

These GPs gave some indication of the possible variations in individual response, but did not consider it appropriate to discuss future problems at this stage. They focused firmly on the present. Any difficulties that might be experienced could be dealt with. It was simply a matter of 'getting it right'. By discussing the use of drugs in these very general terms, concentrating on ironing out any initial problems, GPs could avoid alarming patients and raising doubts as to both the general benefits of the treatment and the efficacy of doctors' own role in its management.

By contrast, two doctors, preferring a more open approach, said they discussed what patients might expect from the medication in some detail. Dr Young, anxious to avoid the uncertainty she felt encouraging unrealistic expectations in her patients might cause, reasoned:

I explain the business about how we can use the drugs, because I think it's quite natural, in a way, for a patient to think 'Well I've got this illness and the doctor's given me the drugs and therefore it will be fixed'. I think you have to bring patients into the idea that things like Sinemet are only useful for a certain length of time. And what you do is support them until the point where they need the drugs, and then you give them the drugs but say they won't actually stop the process. You gradually get them used to the idea that it is a gradual deterioration. Otherwise they're going to get terribly emotionally wound up about the fact that it isn't being fixed.

Dr Smythe also recognized the possibility of causing patients distress if the decreasing efficacy of the treatment over time was not explained. He illustrated the point in a slightly different way:

It's as though they'd been coping with a moderate illness before, a *moderate* disability, and when they start to take levodopa for a period of time they feel great. But when it's not working they're probably no worse than when they started levodopa, but in their minds they feel dreadful because the levodopa's not working. These things often need talking about.

These two GPs viewed patients as rational, autonomous adults, with whom uncertainty could be shared. However, these views were not typical of those of most GPs in the study. The idea of patients logically evaluating the pros and cons of treatment, possibly on different criteria from those of their GPs (see Arluke, 1980; Bury, 1985), was potentially anxiety-laden for most other GPs. It could threaten their role as experts and raise the possibility of non-compliance—situations which several doctors wanted to avoid, as will become apparent later in this chapter.

By placing the rationale for the treatment in broad, general terms, focusing on 'communicating initial problems' (Dr Perlmann) and keeping explanations about any future adjustments 'simple' (Dr Naughton), other doctors hoped to avoid committing themselves to any specific, detailed discussion of the justification for using the treatment which could raise anxieties. While clinical uncertainty, in terms of gauging the effects of the drugs on any one patient, was sometimes acknowledged, it was not presented as being beyond doctors' control. They focused on what could be accomplished in the present and postponed any discussion of the point at which little more could be done clinically. Indeed, they gave no indication that such a point might arise. Let the future take care of itself.

Thus, as the two exceptions indicated above, GPs' policies did vary. But, there was more consensus here than that shown earlier in discussing what to expect. The comparative uniformity of response was even more striking if we consider doctors' ideas about explaining the side-effects of the treatment.

The Side-effects: *'Well, again I wouldn't want to frighten them. I'd say "They might make you drowsy or cause trouble with your waterworks—dryness of the mouth", things like that'*

Explanations about the side-effects of the treatment were treated almost unanimously with caution by GPs in the study—a finding in line with studies of other conditions (see, for example, West, 1976, on epilepsy, and Rosser and Maguire, 1982, on cancer). However, such a consensus might seem surprising given that the medical literature for P.D. patients stresses the importance of information (Stern and Lees, 1982; Godwin-Austen and Hildick Smith, 1982). Duvoisin (1984, pp. 59–60), for example, states: 'I believe it is important that patients know something about their medication. They should understand why they are taking it and what results may be expected. They should be aware of the major side-effects and how we can deal with them.'

The side-effects were almost more difficult for GPs to discuss with their patients than the implications of the illness itself. Doctors with a more cautious approach to information-giving said that they would only talk about the subject if specifically asked. Otherwise, it seemed, they volunteered little. Dr Victor relied on the unpredictability of the drugs' effects to explain his response: 'If I were sure there was some really nasty side-effect I'd say so but I think we're very uncertain.' He did not relay these doubts to his patients. Clinical uncertainty came to serve what Davis (1960) has called 'functional' or 'managerial' ends: medical uncertainty was used to avoid having to make complex decisions about the nature and detail of explanations to be given to individual patients. This absolved doctors from having to confront patients with the anxieties inherent in the limitations of the treatment and, by extension, their own inability to alleviate suffering by purely clinical means.

Other doctors also had reservations. They attempted to give some explanations whilst focusing on the milder end of the spectrum of side-effects. The following comment (Dr Perlmann) was characteristic of this group of GPs:

> I explain it may cause problems in terms of the drugs they take, the anti-cholinergics, the dry mouth and perhaps a little bit of constipation and trouble with urinary retention. The Madopar one can explain that you take it twice a day because it has a certain duration of action. I don't tell them about the on–off effect until they get it.

Dr Black had more explicit concerns on his mind:

> Well, you obviously can't tell people everything about the side-effects and you have to look at the personality of the patient. I mean some people, if you say a drug has a side-effect, they think they're bound to get it, so it may not be wise to say too much. People who are more stoical or sensible I would warn about things like nausea or gastrointestinal upsets so they don't panic if they develop these.

Broad judgements about what patients could and could not cope with again determined what was considered appropriate to say. The 'obviousness' of experience provided the basis for such decision-making, but, as shown in Chapter 2, was largely untested and unquestioned. As Dr Black has indicated, any information was restricted to patients who could be trusted not to react with alarm. Those more easily upset were evidently told little. All round, the problems of the medication were largely underplayed.

Attempts were made to restructure patients' time priorities, emphasizing the present or very immediate future rather than encouraging speculation in the longer term. Dr Perlmann has already shown how doctors preferred to defer explanations, waiting for patients to present with side-effects rather than risk exposing both patient and doctor to a host of unwelcome problems at the outset. Dr Smythe, for instance, said: 'I just wait and see what the patient brings back, if anything. I don't at first talk about on–off effects and what happens after two years.'

Some doctors actively encouraged patients to say what was happening as and when it happened rather than forewarning them of possible future difficulties. Like other doctors, Dr Ellis was reluctant to disclose potentially upsetting information at the start. She reasoned:

> Again I don't give them a list of side-effects they might get. I say to them they'll feel sick *possibly* if they take their tablets on an empty stomach, and to try and take them with or after food and that will reduce the tendency, although there may still be a tendency to feel sick. But if they feel like that to let me know and we'll try and do something about it. We'll supplement it with yet another drug.

Doctors were anxious to stress that medicine had at least some solutions to offer and that these could be tackled together with patients. Such a policy depended for its effectiveness on a close working relationship between patient and doctor and on the provision of arrangements for regular review. Above all, it depended on doctors making space available for patients to ask questions and to voice 'how I feel', when there were often few yardsticks as to how patients should feel, as one patient, reported in Update (1984), indicated. Again the implication was that patients might expect initial difficulties but that these could be ironed out. Any discussion of possible future problems which might be less easily resolved was postponed. Uncertainty was kept in check.

Given the exhortations of the medical literature available for patients and ample evidence from patient studies that '. . . when patients are properly informed about unfamiliar medical interventions and where their anxieties are taken into account, they cope with both better than when they are uninformed and anxious' (Baruch, 1981), why were many of these GPs so reticent?

SOMETHING TANGIBLE ON OFFER: *'Sure, it makes the patients feel better. I don't mean the drugs, but the fact that you can talk of giving something'*

I suggest that the answer lies in the tension between having a treatment available and knowing its problems, especially over time. P.D. is unlike many other chronic illnesses, where palliation rather than direct symptomatic intervention is the most that can be achieved (Robinson, 1988) and where doctors' anxieties about not being able to 'do' anything are often high (Rosser and Maguire, 1982). By contrast, doctors here could do something. However, treatment had problems which they knew, in the current state of medical science, they could probably not resolve.

GPs in the study were divided in their views about the difference having something concrete to offer made to their management. Some felt that it helped, others were ambivalent, and a further group felt that other aspects of management were equally important.

Six GPs felt that the treatment was valuable and helped them in their relationships with patients. For instance, Dr Black said: 'It's the symptomatic relief that matters really'. At the same time GPs acknowledged it made them feel better and 'less inadequate'. Dr Smythe said:

> It makes me feel much better! It makes you feel useful in the sense of being able to give something. I think if you're comparing it to M.S. it's easier to manage than M.S. It's easier to hang a discussion around a change in medication and treatment often, and that for ever to be talking about how someone's continuing to get worse or to have episodes where they feel dreadful where all I can say is 'That must be terrible', it does make you feel better to be able perhaps to give them something which might help.

Giving treatment confirmed doctors in their traditional role of what Rosser and Maguire (1982) refer to as 'mastery through intervention'. This tradition stems from the emphasis given in medical training as well as from the very human desire to solve problems. It gave doctors a sense of doing something positive which outweighed any disquiet about the difficulties in the medication.

Other comments related to the satisfaction experienced in finding their patients 'doing well on treatment' (Drs Victor and Perlmann), or in 'improving their quality of life' (Dr Clements). With this feedback, doctors felt more certain of the value of their intervention.

Perhaps fundamental to the reliance on having something tangible to offer was the desire to preserve patients' hope. Dr Naughton's comments support this. Referring to the explanations given to his patients over the years, he said:

> We need to stress the positive side of management in order to keep hope alive. I'd say 'Fortunately in the last few years there are very good treatments which won't eliminate the problem, but I think we can get it under control'. Again it depends on what they can cope with.... I would say 'There are lots of treatments, there are new things being discovered all the time and we've hardly started yet with these very simple tablets that you're having twice a day. As long as we keep seeing you regularly and you tell me about things, I'm sure we can cope with this illness for a good long time yet.' And I think, by and large, that's true.

These GPs managed uncertainty by encouraging patients to focus on the present while simultaneously inviting them to take a longer view of possible developments in research. Doctors wanted to emphasize what could be done to control the illness with medication now rather than raising possible areas of difficulty. Optimism was vitally important. As Schneider and Conrad (1983) have noted of epilepsy: 'To the extent that doctors believed the drugs were effective they developed great optimism about their ability to treat it.' A similar pattern was evident here.

However, some anxieties were expressed. Dr Threadgold, for instance, thought that the availability of treatment made the patient–doctor relationship both 'easier and more difficult at the same time'. He explained:

> In some ways it makes it all feel comfortable if the doctor is giving the treatment and the patient is taking it and feels better for it. And everyone understands that and feels good about it. Often with Parkinson's you run into a situation where there are problems with side-effects. Whether the overall benefit's good or not, the side-effects are troublesome. And there are feelings of guilt about doing harm, dealing with patients' resentment and resistance. They're taking the treatment that *you* reckon is good for them and *they* reckon isn't.

Balancing costs and benefits in this way caused considerable anxiety. Decision-making which ought to have been easy and routine in fact involved highly complex issues, as he acknowledged when invited to think about it.

Some doctors were also cautious about the value of the treatment, stressing its limitations as a therapy. Dr Richards, for example, thought: 'The thing is you end up in the situation as in so many cases of chronic conditions which you can't do an awful lot about and that's something that makes doctors pretty uncomfortable.' As the medication became less effective over time, GPs felt inadequate at being unable to do anything concrete, a theme which I shall develop in Chapter 6. The ethos of intervention was not lightly discarded. Posner (1977) has shown how doctors continued to treat diabetics with insulin even though some openly admitted that the case for insulin control was far from proven, such was the influence of the curative premise underlying doctors' beliefs. Rosser and Maguire's study (1982) also found doctors reluctant to question the role of physical treatment, even if it impaired the quality of life of patients. The comparative certainty of a curative model of medicine was similarly attractive to many GPs here.

A few doctors were concerned with a much broader interpretation of therapeutic intervention, ideas which Dr Ellis was trying to incorporate into her teaching programme for GP trainers. Similarly, Dr Leadbrough did not think that the medication would make a great difference to her ability to manage patients because:

> . . . you've got all the other things that you're juggling with. I mean we *are* interested very much in the medical side but it's all the other things that make for total fascination really. I mean our job would be quite boring if we were just sticking to the medical side of things.

These GPs wanted to move away from the traditional emphasis on the certainties of biomedical intervention towards embracing the idea of total patient care, of which pharmacological intervention constituted only a part. Treatment was not seen as a 'prop' which absolved them from concentrating on other—perhaps more difficult—aspects of management.

The tension between having something tangible on offer and recognizing the treatment's difficulties and limitations may help to explain the general disinclination to say much to patients about the drugs. The comments of Drs Threadgold and Richards have shown that it could arouse acute unease. The ambiguity shown here raised a further dilemma: namely, the extent to which GPs felt they should control or share the management of their patients' drug regimens.

MEDICAL MANAGEMENT OR SHARED MANAGEMENT?

Over the past decade there has been increasing interest in patient participation, particularly in the management of chronic illnesses, where a measure of responsibility has necessarily to be delegated (Strauss and Glaser, 1975). Managing drug regimens is a twenty-four-hour-a-day task accomplished in the home as much as in a doctor's surgery. Yet studies suggest that participation represents more of a token than any radical change in the balance of power between patient and doctor, and that the issues it raises have been oversimplified (Wiener *et al.*, 1980; Brownlea, 1987). However, participation in its broadest sense involves opening up the agenda with the patient. This could raise anxieties which doctors might prefer to avoid.

Doctors in the study varied in their approach to sharing treatment management decisions with their patients, but distinctions between them were not necessarily consistent with their views on other aspects of communicating with patients.

Doctors Supporting Medical Management: *'They saw the Health Service come in. The doctor did know best. The doctor suddenly had treatments for diseases he never had before and patients don't want to be involved'*

For some GPs, the supervision and management of treatment lay at the heart of medical care and were roles with which they felt at home. Five GPs were correspondingly anxious about the idea of sharing management. Dr Fleming, for example, contrasted his expertise with what he felt were patients' lack of comparable knowledge and inability to evaluate treatment. He considered that:

> Many decisions that have to be made about a patient's illness the patient does not wish to share, just cannot share. . . . The doctor's the person who's been trained to know what the drugs involve and often if you are the type of doctor who says to the patient 'Look, I think this drug could be used in this situation, this is what it might do, these are its potential side-effects, how do you feel about it?' the patient will immediately and quite *rightly* so say 'Well I don't know, doctor. You're the expert, you tell me.' . . . Patients don't want to share. They want doctors to take the responsibility.

The assumption that patients did not wish to share was, as shown in Chapter 2, largely unquestioned and untested. Being in charge not only deflected the anxiety delegation aroused. It also simplified matters: grey areas were eliminated. Drug management was too complicated to be entrusted to 'non-experts'. There were also other considerations which gave doctors momentary pause for thought. Dr Richards reflected:

> I think with levodopa it could be difficult. First of all the patient will tend to get tolerant to it anyway and I think it's probably better not to increase it up too quickly. So in some ways one would want perhaps to keep perhaps a little behind what they want. The other problem is the on–off effect and I think that could be quite confusing. It's quite possible that one might respond by increasing the dosage and afterwards he might overdose by mistake. But again that's something one *could* educate people in, depending on the person I suppose.

On balance, however, the anxieties about patients making mistakes, overdosing or forgetting were more important than the possibility of educating certain patients—raising uncertainty about which patients to choose—in managing the medication. Doctors could not lightly discard traditional ideas of patients as being unable to evaluate treatment and take appropriate action. As far as the treatment was concerned, these GPs appeared to be locked into a model of acute care where being in charge was the natural and obvious response.

Neither Dr Naughton nor Dr Ellis thought that the analogy with diabetes sufficiently justified entrusting the management of P.D. drugs to patients. Dr Ellis thought that the unpredictability of levodopa contrasted unfavourably with the comparatively stable nature of insulin treatment.

Furthermore, Dr Naughton, while welcoming the principle of sharing for younger patients, did not feel that it was suitable for the elderly P.D. patients in his area. 'I think on the whole these are elderly people and my experience of elderly people in this area is that they don't want to be involved with their illness as much as younger people do.' Judgements about age and what the elderly could cope with thus coloured every aspect of management. They dictated not only what was communicated to patients, but also the nature and extent of supervision thought appropriate.

Doctors were uncomfortable with ambiguity. As before, it was handled by reference to the 'obviousness' of experience—what everyone knows the elderly can or cannot cope with. A common working philosophy had distinct advantages. No difficult decisions had to be made as to how much to share, and with whom. However, the adoption of such a house style to suit broad groups of patients precluded an individually tailored approach.

For Dr Quinn, patient sharing in clinical decisions was not a viable proposition. On enquiring, he was surprised that some P.D. patients made daily adjustments to their treatment: 'I don't think they do because that's a very naughty thing to do isn't it.'

Doctors here generally felt that close supervision of their patients' drug regimens was their responsibility as experts, and one which was too risky to be shared. It would raise too many anxieties for both them and, they felt, their patients. Being in charge was an effective means of neutralizing uncertainty.

Doctors Supporting Shared Management: *'Patient autonomy is important and there has to be joint management'*

By contrast, seven other GPs in the study thought that patients should be encouraged to take responsibility—in varying degrees—for the daily management and adjustment of their drugs. While Duvoisin (1984) argues that patients are unable objectively to judge their physical state sufficiently to handle their own medication, these doctors disagreed. Dr Smythe, for instance, talked generally about patients' expertise in handling their own illnesses. He went on: 'As far as the medication's concerned, they can do what they like with it. If their problems carry on they're going to come back and we can discuss if there's anything else we can try.' These doctors respected patients' judgements about both the illness and the treatment. Moreover, the development of patient expertise was a valuable resource for doctors. They could be more assured that they were targeting their management appropriately. Indeed, on-going management relied for its success on patients sharing their accumulating experience of the treatment with their doctors. Patients' knowledge was seen as being complementary, rather than inferior, to that of doctors.

Practical considerations—namely, reducing a workload to manageable proportions—governed Dr Wilkinson's policy. He commented:

> They have to juggle their medication about really. You can't lay down the law and say 'You take your tablets every eighty minutes', or something, because only they know what their requirements are and what the effect is. Not much point for me to monitor them. They can do that.

As far as dealing with any changes in the medication were concerned, he went on: 'Well they usually come and tell me and say "I need more of this", and that's all right.' The unpredictability of the effects of levodopa on any one patient meant that he, too, had to trust his patients' judgements. Clinical uncertainty justified having a more open approach.

Three GPs drew analogies with diabetes to explain the decision to share management. Dr Black thought:

> I mean just like a diabetic should be able to adjust his or her own insulin and should know exactly what his diet and exercise are, I think Parkinson's is very similar. Patients know their own life-style and when it's bothering them and they can take extra when things get troublesome. I think they should be able to do that.

The 'pay-off' in encouraging patients to develop their own expertise was recognized by Dr Clements, who thought that 'it might make people feel a bit more back in control of their own bodies'. In line with her policy on explaining what to expect, she questioned the assumptions of some of her colleagues in classifying the elderly as incompetent. I asked her whether a patient's confusion or memory disturbance might alter her ideas:

> No, I don't think so, unless they've got obvious evidence of mental deterioration. Then you'd be chatting up the spouse. That they would be in on the control of drugs. I think you need to demystify medicine. I think we continually underestimate what patients can understand and do.

—a view well attested to in the literature (see Tuckett *et al.*, 1985).

Comments were too general to reveal the differing levels at which sharing might take place. Nevertheless, it was apparent that the emphasis was on shared management, not the abdication of support. No GP in the study wanted patients to be entirely in control of their own medication. However, sharing decision-making about treatment involved working alongside, rather than being in charge of, patients. These GPs evidently felt that trusting their patients' judgements posed no threat to them.

Indeed, as a strategy, sharing had very positive advantages. It reduced uncertainty all round. GPs felt able to help patients more effectively, with the added advantage of allowing patients to feel in control once more.

SUMMARY AND COMMENT

Handling the treatment was difficult for GPs in the study. Not only were there a number of unknowns about the workings of the drugs themselves, but also doctors were unable to assess accurately how much patients wanted to know about the drugs' side-effects and limitations, and how far patients should be encouraged to take responsibility for the daily management of the treatment. GPs could not know how patients were going to respond, either physically or psychologically.

As before, GPs relied on beliefs and routines to manage the uncertainties to which these issues gave rise. In general, they preferred to give broad statements about what the treatment involved, rather than more specific, detailed explanations. Information about the side-effects was typically bland and low-key: only the milder side-effects were considered appropriate to discuss with patients. Distinctions between doctors were less obvious here than in explaining what to expect of the illness. Again patients were encouraged to focus on the present or the very immediate future. Problems were best dealt with only as and when they occurred. In the short term, the drugs could be relied upon to improve the quality of life for most patients.

As we have already seen in explaining what to expect, softening the information in this way led to fewer misgivings for doctors than confronting patients with the difficulties and limitations of what they had to offer clinically. Given the age of some of their P.D. patients, doctors might be able to spare patients from having to face this situation altogether—a caring policy for Avoiders but intensely frustrating for Seekers. Above all, most doctors were anxious to inspire patients with confidence in the treatment. Although some GPs had serious reservations about its long-term value and preferred a wider interpretation of therapeutic intervention, most found that having a treatment available in itself helped to contain anxieties. The medication gave them something concrete to offer.

Thus, the adoption of such beliefs and routines had important implications for communication: patients who wanted to be protected from the impact of possibly distressing information would be served well by most GPs in the study, but patients seeking more detailed information about short-, medium- and longer-term prospects evidently had to go elsewhere. With a few exceptions, instructions for doctors to be open with information were evidently easier to write about than to apply.

Distinctions between GPs' policies were less consistent over the issue of sharing management where doctors also adopted strategies to manage uncertainty. For some, being in charge minimized the risks and worries of patients forgetting or overdosing. For others, sharing helped them to help their patients. Patients' own experience of the medication was a resource to be tapped.

It might have been expected that those GPs who chose to say little about the illness would also want to be in charge of their patients' medication. This was not always so. GPs who adopted a closed policy to information-giving were also often in favour of sharing management with patients, and vice versa. This may indicate that sharing meant different things to different GPs. It was evident that some doctors were unsure about the various levels on which shared management might take place.

There were two problems here. First, the paucity of information evidently made available to patients suggested that patients were not always equipped with the tools to make sharing a meaningful experience. Participation is not participation if one party lacks the wherewithal to make informed choices. Second, as with explaining information itself, difficulties would arise where patients had different ideas about developing their own expertise from those of their GPs.

It is clear that some of the beliefs and routines developed by GPs to manage the uncertainties of treatment limited the adoption of an individually tailored approach to communication with patients. Fine tuning is as necessary psychologically as it is pharmacologically, as the following chapter will show.

5
The Honeymoon Period—And After

INTRODUCTION

For patients, the availability of treatment raised different concerns. They were confronted with new sources of anxiety which, as I shall show, were experienced and handled very differently from those of the GPs just described. Indeed, some of the uncertainties themselves were different. The drugs had a life of their own which, like the illness itself, required managing if uncertainty was to be controlled.

The worry and distress that managing drug regimens may cause chronically ill patients have only comparatively recently received attention—see the studies of diabetes (Mason, 1985; Kelleher, 1988); epilepsy (Schneider and Conrad, 1983); renal failure (Morgan, 1988); and psoriasis (Jobling, 1988). Anderson and Bury (1988, p. 250) note: 'A medical model of disease is simply inadequate in this task, taking us, as it does, into complex social and emotional areas such as changes in body image, self-medication and growing expertise amongst patients and families themselves.' These areas raise quite different problems from those faced by GPs.

This chapter briefly extends the theme developed in Chapter 3 to include patients' handling of the uncertainties of finding out about the treatment. It then explores some of the wider fears and anxieties raised, and examines the strategies patients evolved for managing them. These revolved around the development of expertise for managing the everyday problems of the medication, particularly strategies of timing and scheduling, where the complex relationship between techniques developed in response to the particular demands of treatment and those which reflected a wider outlook on life emerged clearly. The chapter concludes by looking at the extent to which patients felt their GPs helped them in these tasks.

MISUNDERSTANDINGS AND UNDERSTANDINGS

'I expected to be returned to normal functioning. I expected to be completely fit if I had treatment'

Patients approached the task of acquiring information about the drugs in ways consistent with their abilities, described in Chapter 3, to cope with 'the truth'. However, there was less leeway for manoeuvre with the medication. Only Mrs Franklin was told early on about some of the side-effects of levodopa and no patient was told of its decreasing efficacy over time. A few patients received oblique references to the necessity for periodic juggling to 'get it right'. Evidently, little else was explained other than a broad rationale for using the medication, such as replacing a deficient chemical in the brain (not always the happiest of references: some patients wondered whether this meant that they were 'mentally unbalanced'). Only Miss Norton, on being prescribed levodopa when it first became available, was asked to sign a form saying that she agreed to take medication whose side-effects were unknown. Mrs Quentin and Mr Unwin were also prescribed it early on when little was known of its complications.

Patients said that they had been assured by their doctors that '"we can treat it"' or '"we can control it"'. This assurance allowed some patients to interpret their own situation very positively. Mrs Franklin, for example, thought: '. . . it was just a question of taking a few pills. . . . I assumed that as it got worse I just took more pills, but the idea of the pills losing their efficacy, no.' Mrs Pembridge's understanding was fairly typical of other patients in the study: 'No one actually *said* but I sort of assumed that the medication was always going to be effective. . . . On diagnosis the rheumatologist said "We can treat you" and the way he spoke about treating me I didn't doubt for one moment that it would be successful.' Mrs Mitchell had gone even further, thinking initially that the tablets would 'actually get rid of it. I thought it was a cure, see. But there's no cure.'

The availability of treatment gave those who preferred to let sleeping dogs lie—the Weavers and Avoiders discussed earlier—room to create the best possible interpretation of their case. Particularly when treatment fulfilled the expectations implicitly raised—as it did, several patients commenting favourably on the difference the medication made to their lives initially—anxiety was reduced. The art of reading between the lines worked positively as well as negatively. Reading what one chose to read was an essential survival device for some patients.

'I learnt for myself. It was a journey of discovery and it takes you quite a time to realize that'

However, when the drugs failed to live up to expectations, and side-effects began to occur, patients not surprisingly became anxious. Some patients in the study took things fairly steadily and discovered information from reading or from consulting other sources. Often their own physical response alerted them to the fact that the situation was more complicated than at first anticipated. Mr Vernon, for instance, noted: 'I wasn't told much at first. I learnt from the literature issued by the Society and one learned about them from practical experience. . . . One has the honeymoon period, then gradually you begin to notice that things don't work absolutely perfectly.' He was able to edge his way forward at his own pace. Nothing untoward occurred to force his hand.

By contrast, other patients had a rude awakening. Managing conflicting information was not confined to discovering the implications of having the illness. Mrs Franklin, however, had not yet developed the ability to cope with the frightening picture a different consultant gave her. She recalled:

He said 'There's special medicine out now. Provided you can take it you'll be all right.' I said 'What do you mean "providing I can take it"?'. 'Oh, not everyone can take it. I had one patient who crawled around on the floor and ate his own faeces', which didn't do me any good at all. They told me things which have never happened to me, that one of the common symptoms was seborrhoeic dermatitis and *that* to a female! If I had had it, fine, but to tell me to *expect* it! . . . that was one of the things that had most impact on me. . . . That did frighten me because I'm very vain.

Even years later the sense of outrage was still very strong. At the time she had insufficient knowledge and experience of the effects of the drugs to be able to dismiss the image as not necessarily applying to her. Nevertheless, it was profoundly shocking and upsetting.

Patients who actively searched for information—the Seekers—found that reading between the lines was disturbing. Mr Canning described his growing disquiet: 'My fears were being aroused gradually when further discussion raised the question of different drugs and when the specialist refused to discuss side-effects. . . . I want to *know* what's happening.' Frustration at the lack of response from their doctors affected other patients. Mrs Pembridge described the many occasions when her specialist had similarly refused to discuss the side-effects with her. Moreover, once patients discovered that there were side-effects, there was the additional uncertainty of not knowing what to attribute to what. She went on: 'I feel this very strongly because if I'd been told, I could have distinguished the side-effects from the illness. I do feel it's a right. It's my body, isn't it.'

The situation was particularly difficult for those on multiple drug regimens, such as Mr Jenson. Mrs Jenson was unsure about what could safely be taken together. 'We haven't been told about the side-effects so that you'd *know* what you could combine with what, particularly in J's case with his migraine tablets.' Such uncertainty made coming to terms with the varying symptoms Mr Jenson was beginning to experience particularly difficult.

Thus, discovery of the side-effects and limitations of the treatment was often a shock. New uncertainties were raised. New fears were aroused. As before, information was both a threat and a resource. However, managing uncertainty about what to expect of the drugs seemed more difficult than coming to understand the implications of the illness itself. Patients were not accustomed to question what doctors prescribed. Nor were they familiar with, or able to obtain, details of the pharmacological properties of the drugs. They mostly worked in the dark, so that only those pursuing 'softly, softly' strategies were relatively free from anxiety on this score at the outset. Doctors were evidently not to be pressed. However, once patients discovered that there were side-effects, most wanted to know what they were. They became Seekers. Within limits, patients felt they could *do* things about the drugs. Unlike the illness itself, drugs were amenable to human control. Therein, as patients were to discover, lay the potential for managing uncertainty.

BEING ON TABLETS

The prevailing medical view that 'medication is something doctors prescribe and patients take' (Schneider and Conrad, 1983) has rarely addressed the meanings which drugs have for patients. Concern with compliance has obscured the fact that patients actively evaluate their regimens for effectiveness and compatibility with their life-styles, and make decisions accordingly (Arluke, 1980; Bury, 1985).

Being on tablets for life was often distressing for patients. Three main themes emerged in patients' accounts which aroused anxiety: the unpredictability of the treatment itself and its effects on life-style; dependence; and medical complacency.

(1) The unpredictability of the effects of the drugs heightened anxiety and frustration for some patients. The inability to make even short-term plans made life erratic and consequently upsetting. Four patients commented on previous or current periods of instability when the variability of the treatment made living a near-normal life impossible. Mrs Richards said of her husband: 'The medication sometimes worked and it sometimes didn't. . . . And sometimes in the evenings he had such *restless* periods and was wretched. . . . There were times even after taking the extra pill it didn't work.' Mr Richards said: 'You can't manage and control your life on that basis.' The regimen was difficult enough to manage at the time. He thought that it would have been totally incompatible with a previous working life characterized by irregular hours and meals.

The intrusiveness of the regimen into patients' lives was also disturbing. Feelings ranged from varying degrees of frustration and anger at the detailed monitoring the regimen required—as Mr Grenville put it, 'Spontaneity is off'—or the responsibility involved in ensuring that pills were ordered, collected and taken at the right time (Mrs York of her husband), to feeling completely taken over by the medication. Mrs Pembridge acknowledged: 'It runs me. It's running my life. I've got to take medicine at different times to enable me to do things. It's not a case of "take one tablet a day".' She had slept through the alarm on the day I was due to see her: 'First when I looked at my watch and it was 9.15 I was horrified. I can't just jump out of bed and put my clothes on, can I? My first thought was "I must get those tablets down me".' Pills dominated her life—a state of affairs which distressed her. However, it was only through such minute attention to the demands of the medication that she was able to feel at least partly in control. As we shall see, patients' attempts to develop some expertise were often a direct response to the unpredictability and intrusiveness of the regimen on their lives.

(2) Second, most patients disliked being dependent on drugs. Being on tablets for the rest of their lives was often a blow. Pill-taking was seen as 'unnatural', for emergencies only. Several patients had prided themselves on 'never taking a pill in my life, not even aspirin' (Mr Unwin). To be told 'Well, you'll have to get used to it' (Mr Canning's consultant) detracted from patients' autonomy. It seemed that they forfeited their ability to be in charge. Mr Richards said:

> I'm very dependent on them . . . I don't like it. They're the very first I've ever had on which I've been dependent. . . . It's the very practical feeling I have from having taken them. You can feel the change coming over in the process of an hour. . . . If I got up in the morning and found I didn't have any and couldn't see a source, I'm not sure what I'd do.

The fear of dependence escalating out of control was illustrated by Mr Canning. He saw himself trapped in a continuing spiral of drugs, each new drug counteracting the adverse side-effects of the previous one:

> There's one devastating paragraph in the black and white book [Godwin-Austen, 1984] which says 'You take levodopa for this disease and then this is likely to cause constipation so you take another drug to deal with that, and another drug for the depression side of it'. So you're taking drugs to deal with maybe six conditions. I worked it out and I thought you'd have to take a little stopwatch and say 'It's pill-time'.

The dread of dependence and the attendant loss of being in charge of one's own body was profoundly disturbing.

(3) Third, three patients found the complacency with which they felt the medical profession regarded the treatment worrying. Mrs Jenson fretted: 'I just feel they're only doing what they want. They've got their pet projects.

There's no urgency there. There's no "For God's sake, *do* something".' Mr Grenville developed the theme:

> I feel very strongly that the myth of the wonder drug, levodopa, has been perpetuated continually in the sense that the impression has been given that there is a drug which has a few side-effects which have been worked out in research and the answer to the side-effects is just around the corner. The majority of research tends to be channelled in this direction, perfecting the administration of the drug, whereas an alternative view . . . may be to accept that drugs are part of the answer but that a considerable contribution towards managing the illness could be made which doesn't entail the use of drugs. . . . It gives a public impression that here's an illness that can now be discarded as presenting problems by people suffering from it, because although not a cure a remedy is now available for it.

When patients knew the side-effects and limitations of the current drug therapy and felt that there was little incentive for medical research to pursue other avenues of enquiry, future prospects looked bleak. Mr Canning could only look on helplessly at the current media coverage of AIDS and wish that some of that urgency could be channelled into finding a remedy for P.D.

Not only were patients' views about being on tablets more elaborate and sophisticated than the traditional medical focus on compliance has suggested; patients' feelings about the drugs raised very real anxieties and fears.

This section has emphasized the difficulties of the drug regimen. It is also important to mention patients' positive feelings. Most patients in the study felt that the treatment improved their condition, at least for an initial period. Mrs Quentin, for instance, described with wry amusement her relief that the treatment worked. Her consultant had simply handed her a prescription without further explanation:

> When you look back on it he said so very little and I thanked him very nicely for stopping the tremor! Because I'd never known it stopped before and I was delighted. I didn't ask what the tablets were about. I suppose it was stupid of me, but all I could think of was they stopped the shaking in my hands.

Three patients were confident that it was 'just a question of time' before medical research produced 'the answer', were less perturbed by dependence on drugs and did not find their daily administration so intrusive.

When things started to go wrong, however, fears and anxieties were aroused. I shall explore patients' attempts to manage the drug regimen as a means of gaining some purchase over what was happening.

ROOM FOR MANOEUVRE OR PLAYING IT BY THE BOOK?

As the previous chapter stressed, the medical literature for the lay person emphasizes the importance of patients following their doctors' instructions, although attitudes towards strict timetabling have been modified recently (Thompson, 1987). Perhaps the greatest anxiety for patients came with the growing realization that they knew as much as, if not more than, their doctors about the effects of the treatment on *them*. Moreover, their doctors depended on this subjective assessment to 'get it right'. Mr Dempsey's consultant put it to him: '"So long as you don't overdose yourself, give anything a try. It's in your hands".' This left patients in a dilemma. On the one hand, they were urged to conform to the traditional image of the passive patient and to comply with instructions; on the other, they were encouraged to experiment with doses and timing, thus introducing an additional element of uncertainty into their lives. Studies of diabetics (Mason, 1985; Posner, 1988) and polio patients with post-respiratory difficulties (Locker and Kaufert, 1988) have pointed out this contradiction. Alexander (1980, pp. 317–318), in his study of patients on haemodialysis, noted that patients are simultaneously seen as incompetent and sick '. . . yet they are ultimately expected to learn to administer the entire treatment. . . . Compliance, conformity, co-operativeness, and doing what one is told are exceedingly different from trying to mobilize self-sufficiency and independence of decision . . . where the required resources for such action are controlled by others.' Yet little attention has been paid to the task of easing the transition of patients between the two positions.

The situation was fraught with uncertainty for patients in the study. Such uncertainty required managing. It was handled in two ways: (1) Patients learned to adjust the drugs on an everyday basis themselves, with varying degrees of supervision from consultant and/or GP, and developed timing strategies to facilitate this. This gave them confidence and alleviated anxiety. (2) More rarely, patients handed over control to the experts. The responsibility was too overwhelming. In practice, patients often moved in and out of the two positions as they gained confidence, or, conversely, as they lost their way when crises arose which necessitated a return to close medical regulation.

'You realize how to take them in a way that suits you. You've got to find out for yourself. You can't rely on doctors doing it for you'

Mr Vernon illustrated how he had resolved the situation over time:

Mr Vernon: One consultant I visited said 'play around with the dosages' and the GP has said something very similar. 'Take four or five a day, four or five, it's within your discretion.'
R.P.: How do you feel about being given that responsibility?
Mr Vernon: All I can say is that it doesn't worry me. I guard against the temptation to build up the dosage. And my GP understands this and he has

confidence in me. He's often said 'You know as much about it as I do. Shall we try this or that?'

Patients thus discovered that the onus for handling the daily management of the drugs lay on them. Confidence in their judgement came with experience over time. Patients mostly valued the responsibility, as it gave them an opportunity to exercise some control over their enforced dependence on medication. Mrs Franklin, for example, was pleased with the instructions her consultant had given her GP: 'They say in their letter "This lady is intelligent, she knows what she's doing, will adjust her own dose".'

Success in handling this largely unexpected responsibility depended on patients' ability to develop timing and scheduling strategies to make the most of life when they could. Timetabling was important in enabling patients to be in charge. Mrs Franklin described her work: 'I timetable my day. I rearrange my day and my pills so that I can get the utmost when I need it. I control it to that extent.'

Mr Dempsey and Mr Grenville had worked out sophisticated regimens which gave them maximum scope to engage in activities they valued. Mr Dempsey was intent on preserving his social life, regularly attending tea dances in the hope of meeting a second wife. He scheduled his pill-taking around his social engagements:

> The way my life was going I've got to have some bad times and I've got to have some good times. If I could sort out the good times when I could go out or be taken out with friends, go for a pint or have a bit of social life that was great. If I suffer for it in the morning when I'm on me own that's too bad. I'm willing to put up with that. . . . It all comes back to the fact of juggling around to get the pleasure I can. I know that out of twenty-four hours I can get, say, four or six hours of good time. So my day isn't a twenty-four-hour day, it's a four- or a six-hour day. . . . If I've got six or eight hours on me own and six or eight hours with someone else, I want the six or eight hours good with the other people, I don't care about the others.

Other patients made less detailed calculations, but the principle was similar.

Managing the regimen also *took* time in the sense that patients had to postpone activities until the medication took effect. Mr Unwin described his daily disappointments. He had to wait to be in charge once more.

> I get very frustrated. Especially about an hour before I have the tablets. I'm getting ready for them too early. Getting impatient for the relief. . . . I wait to take the pills and then I know that in a couple of hours I can move about. I'm waiting on the pills. Everything's waiting on the pills.

Waiting generated tension and impatience. Yet Mr Unwin knew that relief was at hand and that he would be able to carry on again. He managed the difficult wait. Such strategies represented very practical attempts to control the specific problems presented by the drug regimen. They also reflected broader outlooks on life: patients did not give up easily.

Most patients in the study adopted a policy of cramming activities into those parts of the day when they were at their best, even if, as in the case of Mr Irving and Mr York, these were only small segments of time during the day and were in themselves not reliable. Controlling the medication in these ways—being responsible for its day-to-day management and acquiring some expertise in handling its unpredictabilities—was important in managing the fears and anxieties which being on tablets aroused. It gave patients a tool with which to combat feelings of helplessness. They were not passive patients.

'I want him to play it by the rules'

For other patients this unexpected responsibility represented a threat. It left patients casting around helplessly for guidance which was evidently not forthcoming. Where were the rules? Mr Canning for example, said:

> It's not a question of their permitting me to adjust. There's an *absence* of suggestions as to what might be the right amount. . . . There doesn't seem to *be* any advice. Nobody has ever said, 'Oh yes, you need *x* number of pills per day'. It's always 'Try this and see if it works'. Nobody's ever said 'We'll test this and we'll test that to see if you need *x* or *y* number of pills'.

In the absence of clear instructions and a 'scientific' basis for proceeding, Mr Canning tested the drugs himself, increasing or decreasing the dosage to see whether they were doing any good. However, he was too frightened to drop them altogether. The inability to find reliable yardsticks against which to assess his own response to the treatment was profoundly disturbing. He was unused to—and unprepared for—such a situation. The uncertainty was unnerving. Similarly, Mr Richards, who had been 'given permission' to vary his dosage from eight to nine tablets a day exploded: 'I want a specialist to get hold of me and shake me and say "Here's a regime. Now go away and *stick* to it".' He was at a loss to handle the leeway he had been given. Moreover, being in charge was at variance with his previous experience of patienthood for a recent thyroid operation, where, perforce he felt, he had surrendered control to his doctors. The contrast between the experience of chronic and acute illnesses emerged sharply. The latter lent themselves to swift, confident decision-making by doctors; the former turned out to be full of uncertainties.

Patients often alternated between periods of medical and shared regulation over time. At the outset, as expected, patients complied with instructions to the letter, unaware of the trial-and-error process involved. Mr Mitchell, for example, took his tablets 'exactly as I've been prescribed them', carefully supervised by his wife.

Over time, things often changed. Mrs Pembridge, for instance, although altering her dosage in a minor way to suit her needs earlier, subsequently had a crisis; she was dried out in hospital and a new drug regimen was instigated. Under these circumstances, uncertainty was rekindled. She wanted very specific guidance:

> I want all the 't's crossed and the 'I's dotted. I don't know enough about what goes with what to muck about. I want him [consultant] to tell me what he wants and I'll stick to the letter. . . . He's got all the experience with other patients. He knows far more than I ever will. I can't be on my own with these drugs.

Finally Mrs York was unable to cope with the responsibility for her husband's medication. She relied totally on both consultant and GP, although support was not always seen to be forthcoming. The fears aroused by being in charge were too threatening.

COMMENT

Patients were thus ill-prepared to find themselves responsible for evaluating the treatment and handling the daily management of the drugs. However, most responded to the challenge. Being in charge increased their self-confidence and gave them the feeling of being in control again. However, other patients were reassured only when their doctors took charge. Where this did not happen, it caused great distress. It cannot be assumed that liberal ideas about sharing medical treatment decisions were always welcomed. It was very much an individual matter, and had to be addressed as such if uncertainty was to be minimized.

PATIENTS' VIEWS OF THEIR GPs

For patients in the study, all but three of whom had seen a consultant at some time during their illness, advice on drugs was seen primarily as a consultant's province. Nine patients thought that their GP was inexperienced in drug management. This meant that patients relied heavily on their consultants for detailed adjustment and overall practical help, but were reluctant to 'bother them' with deeper worries about the medication. Patients often fell between two stools—between the consultant and the GP, neither catering adequately for the complexity of patients' needs—as Maguire's (1984) study of cancer patients showed. It is a pattern characteristic of many chronically ill patients (Gerson and Strauss, 1975).

The Mechanics Only

'Just for prescriptions'
Although patients often badly needed a GP's help, many patients felt that their GP was unwilling to get involved in this area. Mr and Mrs Mitchell thought that a GP would be 'Talking about it, telling you what to expect and what will happen and what all the tablets are for'. Mrs Mitchell:

'Instead of just dishing out prescriptions they should try and explain to you.'

Similarly, Mr Dempsey found that his GP refused to take any interest in, or responsibility for, his medication, always referring him back to the consultant. He would have welcomed the chance to talk with a GP who he thought was sufficiently familiar with the drugs to allay his fears, although under the circumstances referral to his consultant was considered appropriate. He wanted to talk at two levels. 'If I go and see my GP and say to him "I'm having it a bit rough at the moment, do you think I can alter the medication?" he says "You'd better get in touch with the hospital, I don't know enough about it". He won't give me any indication whatsoever about altering the dosage or anything.' His GP did not respond to the underlying anxiety that the remark 'having it a bit rough' conveyed. Moreover, consulting one health professional about differing aspects of the same problem was discouraged. While Mr Dempsey respected an honest admission of inexperience, he saw the apparent unwillingness to remedy this as a rebuff. As a result, he could not broach worries about both the technical and the emotional aspects of drug management.

Lack of liaison between consultant and GP again featured in patients' accounts. Mr and Mrs Jenson had visited their GP in an effort to get things straightened out. Mrs Jenson commented:

> The GP does agree to cut down on the migraine tablets and he's said 'Right, we'll cut the 118 [Dixarit] out'. And J. goes to Dr X and says 'I'm out of 118s' and comes back with a bottle full. So there's no tie-up between one doctor and another. And that makes me furious. . . . It made me feel very bitter towards the GP because when J. went back from taking the two to the one he was a different person.

Her frustration at the lack of co-operation and ensuing uncertainty was compounded when the GP telephoned, following Mr Jenson's bowel operation, to query the drugs he was taking. She fumed: 'What he's taking should be on the *notes*.' There were administrative, as well as physical and psychological, problems to contend with.

Lack of appreciation of what being on tablets meant to patients also had important outcomes for future patient–GP relationships. Both Mr Canning's previous GP and his consultant had been pressing him to take antidepressants. This was no solution in his eyes. He said:

> I mean in the book [Godwin-Austen, 1984], it says you ought to let the doctor manage your prescribing. Well, frankly, I'm up against a specialist who seems to be pill-minded. . . . I don't know what the devil I'd have been taking if I'd left it up to them. I would be taking Amitriptyline now and drugging myself up to the eyeballs for depression.

He felt that neither GP nor consultant appreciated the fear of dependence and loss of control reliance on drugs represented to him.

In these circumstances, patients used their GPs simply as pick-up points for their monthly prescriptions. It left a rather bleak picture of patients struggling to make sense of a regimen that was often unpredictable and sometimes frightening. Managing the uncertainties of the drugs needed more regular personal attention than three- or six-monthly appointments with a consultant. Here the delicate task of attuning themselves to patients' changing needs for information and support—which GPs were ideally placed to do—was not even on the agenda. The relevance of these patients' GPs to their lives as P.D. patients was marginal.

A Friend Indeed

'You'd be fighting on your own without your GP'
The contrast between these experiences and those of the five patients who found their GPs knowledgeable and helpful about the drugs could not have been stronger. A joint partnership between patient, GP and consultant was the essence of a good, caring relationship for these patients. Anxieties were at a minimum, with GPs readily accessible and willing to discuss problems when they occurred and to respect the meanings being on drugs held for patients. Mrs Quentin, for instance, said:

> If I thought I wanted the dosage increased further, I'd go and tell him [the GP] and we'd discuss it. And the thing is you wouldn't be afraid to go to him. He would listen to you, although I know he's not a great one for tablets. But then he'd want me to go back to the neurologist.

Unlike Mr Dempsey, Mrs Quentin never felt rebuffed at the referral, as her GP always took time and care to explain things before she went and supported her on her return.

Both Mr Vernon and Miss Norton had found their GPs supportive when they underwent brain surgery (a procedure known as stereotactic surgery, which was performed fairly often before the advent of levodopa). Miss Norton wrote: 'This GP, he gave me strength and reassurance. . . . It was he who encouraged me to have the operation. He told me it was the only thing that could help me.' Despite her subsequent loss of speech, she did not regret her decision. A warm relationship with her GP was sustained over the following twenty years, until his death.

The one instance in the study where a patient's GP had adjusted the medication himself had left a lasting impression on Mr and Mrs Unwin. Mrs Unwin described what happened:

> He was marvellous about three years ago when U. got worse. He was here nearly every week trying to change them over and balance them. He went from May right through to Christmas, nearly every week, and then every two weeks. And then he said 'That's the best I can do. Now he's steady. Get your mobility in the morning.' He'd juggled the tablets right the way through.

Their GP was both sympathetic with their underlying disquiet and experienced with the workings of the drugs. Mr and Mrs Unwin trusted him and respected his judgement. Anxieties were allayed.

This evidence suggests that a joint partnership between patient and GP, and, in most cases, between patient, GP and consultant, could work and effectively reduce patients' worries. Again a firm knowledge base, or the willingness to develop one, was vitally important, as was the demonstration of care and concern. These five patients were generally content that everything that could be done had been done and that no effort had been spared in alleviating their worries.

SUMMARY AND COMMENT

Jobling (1988, p. 229) has noted that drug regimens as well as being 'part of "the solution"' are also 'part of "the problem"'. The uncertainties patients confronted here were of a different order from those which concerned GPs: namely, discovering the side-effects and limitations of the drugs, and finding that they themselves were 'the experts' in learning how to use them to their best advantage.

When problems arose and patients found that there were side-effects to contend with, they were often shocked and upset. In the same way that they came to understand the implications of the illness, the discovery that the drugs were not so simple as patients sometimes anticipated was a gradual process for some, less so for others. Most patients were given little information other than a broad rationale for the treatment which initially allowed Weavers and Avoiders to build an optimistic picture of their own case. However, when Seekers were unable to pin their doctors down, they found the task of reading between the lines intensely frustrating. A closed policy to communicating information raised patients' anxieties rather than allaying them.

Patients perhaps felt the greatest sense of foreboding when they realized that they knew as much as their doctors about the effects the treatment had on them. There was little preparation for such a discovery. Several patients had had acute illnesses where—quite appropriately, they felt—the doctor had been in charge. When they found that treatment in a chronic illness such as P.D. could not be managed in the same way, this often conflicted with their ideas of what medicine was about. The repeated comment '"Only you can know what it feels like; you know best what your body tells you"' when patients felt they did not made the situation thoroughly unnerving.

Moreover, the very fact of being on tablets for life often upset patients. Most had grown up before the pharmacological explosion of the 1950s and were unused to the idea of 'a pill for every ill'. Yet drugs were, I believe, a more readily accessible target for anxiety than the illness. Medication was under human control rather than being 'an act of God'. Something could be done about the drugs.

Patients tried to impose order on this new experience by developing expertise in handling the everyday timing and scheduling of dosages and in gaining experience about using the drugs in a way that best suited them. They gained confidence in judging for themselves when they needed changes in their medication. These practical techniques were incorporated into a wider repertoire of skills which reflected their broader outlook on life. Over time, most patients enjoyed this unexpected responsibility. It allayed some of the deeper anxieties raised by the prospect of lifelong dependence on medication, and helped them to regain a sense of being in charge of their own bodies once more. For others, however, the situation was profoundly threatening. They were not always able to cope with the demands involved. When crises arose and where support and guidance were not forthcoming, a few patients were at a loss. Liberal ideas about shared decision-making did not suit all comers at all stages of the illness.

Patients who did not have supportive relationships with their GPs often felt anxious, frustrated and depressed. These patients' stories left one with a feeling of missed opportunities. If only a GP had been there at that particular moment, so much anxiety and suffering might have been avoided. For most patients in the study, the role of their GP in treatment management was marginal (at variance with what GPs in the study felt they could do). Patients thought their GPs were often reluctant to become involved and were inexperienced in handling the technicalities. In these situations, doctors were evidently in no position to engage with their patients' needs. Where consultants were on the scene, they tended to be pivotal, but most patients felt that the expression of worries and anxieties was outside their province. They were often stranded in a no-man's-land between consultant and GP, where anxiety was high. Conversely, the crucial difference a supportive and knowledgeable GP made to the lives of other patients in the study indicated what could be achieved here. These latter patients felt at ease, knowing that any worries could readily be attended to. They felt responded to as individuals with unique needs and expectations. Uncertainty was reduced.

Above all, patients' anxieties about the drug regimen were intensely personal, requiring as much psychological as physiological adjustment. A standardized response with which some GPs in the study seemed to operate was quite inappropriate for their needs. The importance of individualized care in managing the uncertainties of the whole P.D. experience has been a recurrent theme and one to which I shall return in Chapter 7. First, I shall explore GPs' responses to managing the fundamental questions raised by dealing with their P.D. patients.

6
Detachment or Empathy?

INTRODUCTION

The fundamental human concerns raised by the onset of a chronic illness such as P.D. can present the GP with profound difficulties. Many of us choose to ignore such questions until personally faced with situations of loss, bereavement or incapacitating illness. GPs, however, at all stages of their careers, are squarely confronted with questions of how much to take on, of how far to go in opening themselves to patients' distress. The questions demand a response to human suffering. This may create deep fears and anxieties in GPs themselves, as this chapter will show.

The Royal College of General Practitioners' motto *Cum Scientia Caritas* may be translated as caring with knowledge. Caring is for 'the whole person'. But this may mean quite different things to different GPs. As Wilson (1986) notes: '. . . as in all aspects of General Practice, the GP can do as much or as little as he wants for the individual patient'. While freedom is a challenge, it also admits a great ambiguity over what is a legitimate role for the GP to play in this wider area of his/her work. Likewise, the means of evaluating success or failure in the chosen role are also more elusive.

Several studies have shown the fear and role ambiguity which GPs face when brought too close to the suffering of cancer patients and the terminally ill (Maguire, 1984, 1985; Still and Todd, 1986), and the difficulties medical students experience in coping with patients' distress (Ridsdale, 1987). Maguire *et al.* (1986) and Walker (1988) have also shown the reluctance of doctors to ask questions which might reveal a host of problems with which they feel ill-equipped to deal. However, comparatively little attention has been paid to the ways GPs manage what Hasler (1985) calls 'the very stuff of general practice'.

This chapter first explores how GPs in the study thought they handled the special difficulties which arose from three aspects of P.D.: its progressive nature, the inability of doctors to cure it and, in some cases, a breakdown in normal methods of communication. It then focuses in more detail on two complementary areas of 'feeling work' (Strauss *et al.*, 1985) which highlighted how far GPs responded to patients' distress. These were the exploration of patients' fears and anxieties, and the ease or discomfort they felt with listening to or just being together with patients. I shall examine the main strategies GPs adopted to deal with any feelings of inadequacy or helplessness—principally by the use of time, pacing and scheduling. The issue is one of professional involvement: how GPs struck balances between detachment and empathy as a means of coming to terms with the uncertainties of handling this delicate area of work. Finally I shall draw out the implications of my findings for communication between patient and doctor.

Distinctions between doctors were again often blurred. Nevertheless, some patterns emerged. All GPs in the study claimed that caring, however defined, played an important part in their work with patients. Dr Arlen saw the task as:

> . . . total patient care, listening, supporting, keeping in touch. . . . If people talk about their relationships and how they're feeling, if they go on talking about them, they actually begin to listen to what they're saying and it will begin to come out. It's a bit like an onion skin. A bit comes off and then you get down to the next bit, and I think just encouraging people to talk about it and how they feel about it is the best way of dealing with it.

The special difficulties in applying this principle to P.D. patients emerged from a consideration of specific aspects of the illness.

DOWN TO BASICS: PROGRESSION, INCURABILITY AND 'THE P.D. FACE'

'It's a progressive illness . . .'

First, P.D. presents doctors with the task of sustaining the quality of care through a series of gradually deteriorating personal and family crises over a long time-span. There is no immediate end in sight. In this way chronic illness is perhaps more difficult to manage than caring for the terminally ill—or, as Dr Perlmann put it, P.D. is itself a long-drawn-out terminal illness. Some evidence for this was supplied by five doctors with more flexible approaches to management. Dr Ogilvie for instance, said: 'It becomes progressively harder to look after the patient in a caring, humanitarian way.' Though in every other way Dr Smythe considered that he was receptive to patients' distress, he found the long-term caring for P.D. patients a strain. He acknowledged frankly: 'I think that's something I don't cope with that well.' Dr Clements talked of a P.D. patient she had looked after: 'I also remember the feeling, and I think you have to be aware of it, when you actually say "I've run out of sympathy". It's only a temporary patch. It's just that you've run out of steam and haven't another suggestion to make.' Doctors were uncertain where to go next, how they could best help when it seemed they had tried everything there was to try.

While I did not directly compare attitudes to chronic illness and terminal care, which might be thought to have many elements in common, it appeared that 'securing a good death'—which several doctors mentioned spontaneously as a source of satisfaction—perhaps had more in common with handling acute illnesses. The sheer staying power necessary to sustain the quality of care over time in a chronic illness often taxed emotional resources to the limit.

Equally, the satisfactions in caring for the chronically ill were more elusive. Dr Richards thought: '. . . you have to dig deeper to get the rewards in chronic illness, to try harder. They're not easy to treat. You've got to put in more effort.' There were no immediately obvious benefits from their intervention.

'It's nice when they get better, isn't it'

Second, coming to terms with the inability to cure P.D. was also a source of anxiety for some GPs in the study. Several doctors mentioned this regretfully. Dr Perlmann, for instance, commented: 'One of the difficult things about medicine is accepting that people don't get better.' This exposed not only doctors' own limitations as practising professionals—the tools with which they were well equipped were not always appropriate— but also the constraints of modern medicine itself. Doctors often felt inadequate.

The 'fun' or 'buzz', as Dr Naughton described it, in making people better was illustrated several times. Dr Young mused: 'Acute illness is good fun. . . . One of the nice things about being a doctor is that you can fix things. If you can't then it's harder because you've got to come to terms with the fact that you can't fix things.' One gained the impression that sometimes discussion of P.D. was accompanied by nostalgia for the comparative certainties of acute medicine, even though GPs acknowledged that certainty was not a realistic goal for much of their work. Dr Naughton put it trenchantly: 'I think general practice mainly is chronic illness and if you don't like it then you shouldn't be doing it.'

'There's a tendency with P.D., as with all handicapped people, to suddenly become a non-person because of the way the illness can express itself'

Third, often the basic structures of communication were deficient or lacking, leaving doctors feeling frustrated and helpless. Some aspects of P.D., particularly speech deterioration, memory impairment and the loss of facial expression, affect patients' ability to respond. They deprive the listener of important cues such as turn-taking and feedback. Many GPs commented on this. Dr Perlmann, for instance, noted:

> One of the problems of Parkinson's patients is that it's actually very difficult to empathize with them, because the Parkinson's face provides one with little feedback. And that makes it difficult for an observer. One can do what one has to but one doesn't get the cues that one can respond to. It makes it more difficult to discuss things with Parkinson's patients.

GPs were uncertain of the benefits of their services when the usual basis for evaluation was absent. Under these circumstances it was often difficult to maintain a close relationship with patients. Analogies with the deaf and hard of hearing (Pinder, 1983) and other chronic conditions such as stroke (Brocklehurst *et al.*, 1981) spring readily to mind. Goffman (1963) has vividly described the discomfort 'communicative incompetence' arouses in our culture. We place a high premium on the ability to be articulate. Those who are deficient in this respect tend to be marginalized, if not actively stigmatized (Baker and Pinder, 1989). GPs in the study evidently experienced the same unease as lay persons.

I now turn to two crucial areas of management: exploring patients' fears and anxieties, and the extent to which GPs thought listening, or just being there—where the risks of exposing themselves to patients' basic human concerns were high—were necessary and legitimate parts of their role. The capacity of doctors to respond to such problems is, I believe, a good indication of their ability to deal with the anxieties which an open approach raises.

EXPLORING FEARS AND ANXIETIES: *'I've got a responsibility to facilitate that for them'*

Several doctors in the study thought it important to encourage their P.D. patients to express their troubles—at least in principle. Dr Ogilvie, for example, felt: 'By asking broad, open questions, I would hope to lead a patient into telling me what he was feeling within himself. I'm trying to decide what they feel about their condition. That's top of the list.' As a trainee, he had not yet been exposed to the full demands of general practice. However, when interviewed, he felt able to carry out these ideas with the number of patients for whom he was responsible. Moreover, he thought that encouraging patients to express their fears helped them to come to terms with their situation. Dr Dandridge, with long experience, considered that it was an essential ingredient of her work that her P.D. patients 'should feel free to unburden themselves'.

Some GPs thought that exploring patients' deeper feelings about the illness was part of their repertoire of interviewing skills. Dr Smythe explained: 'It's part of the consultation technique that I use in that I try and find out what their fears are. I always ask them what's gone through their minds, have they anything they're particularly worried about with the symptoms they're having.'

Nevertheless, some indication of the tensions and anxieties which such receptivity posed was illustrated by Dr Clements. She paced herself according to the demands of time, the necessity for personal survival and her commitment to openness. She was thus able to strike a balance between empathy and detachment which allowed her to respond to patients' distress without being overwhelmed by anxiety herself:

> I think with neurological conditions, there are other aspects of life you've got to keep exploring, or presenting the opportunity for people to express their fantasies, because they're going to be much more recurrent, aren't they? About fault, about mental deterioration, about dependence and how quickly it may come. . . . But I think you *can* give time, ten minutes, quarter of an hour. Say someone's distressed. I think in twenty minutes you can either find out do they need psychotherapy, a psychiatrist or whatever, or at least sort out the priorities.

At the same time she had her eye firmly fixed on what she called 'the ultimate ball game'. She continued:

> I think to a certain extent the sheer numbers in general practice end up by protecting you. They provide a safety valve. Like if you get overwhelmed by someone's distress in the surgery you actually *have* to be very business-like because there are ten others and they cough to let you know they're there!

While adopting a flexible time-schedule allowed her to be sensitive to her patients' needs, she was also aware of her personal limitations. She could not contain more than a certain amount of distress and relied on the pressure of numbers to keep things under control.

These GPs were aware of, and had learnt to deal with, patients' distress and the anxieties it raised in themselves. Like all GPs in the study, they contained the anxiety which increasing opportunities for discussion might produce by keeping a watchful eye on their personal stamina and by a judicious, but flexible, distribution of their time. At the same time, they saw the relief of distress as one of the most important parts of general practice, one to be shared *with* patients as far as possible. Doctors did not want to leave their patients floundering on their own. Sharing was seen as part of the process of helping patients adjust to the illness and of managing both their patients' and their own deeper feelings.

The question of time dominated the thoughts of most GPs in the study. Horobin (1983) has distinguished between time as a 'real' constraint in general practice, in the sense of achieving a given volume of work within a set time span, and its use as 'an account', determining which patients can be coped with in any one period of time. A GP who has time for X but insufficient time for Y is giving X priority. Value judgements, of necessity, are being made. The way doctors in the study used time as an 'account' had a major impact on the position they took in resolving the empathy–detachment equation.

Dr Ellis was one of the few doctors in the study to appreciate how GPs' attitudes to time both were shaped by and in turn shaped their ideas about the value of encouraging patients to express their distress. She exploded when I raised the issue:

DR ELLIS: The poor overworked doctor! It's a load of rubbish. It's a myth. We work as hard as we want to. There's nobody here who's grossly overworked. I mean you ought to go and work in Nigeria and see five hundred patients a day. Then you're overworked. This business about pressure is partly created from inside.
R.P.: What do you think doctors can do about it?
DR ELLIS: They can rethink it.
R.P.: That means turning time upside down, doesn't it?
DR ELLIS: Yes, but is there any reason why we shouldn't? I think we're obsessed by time. And we create pressures inside ourselves because of time.

In reorganizing her work to give time to patients' distress, she illustrated the way it rested as much on judgements about the 'proper' use of time, which were amenable to change, as on the ticking of the clock. She, too, was ready to accept the uncertainties—of keeping others waiting, of disrupting her own routine, and, most importantly, of exposing herself to the pain of others—which a flexible attitude to time entailed. Within limits she wanted to be involved.

However, other doctors had misgivings about the issue. Dr Threadgold said of one of his terminally ill cancer patients: 'I'd like to go and talk to him but I know I'd be there three-quarters of an hour and I can't do it.' Referring to his everyday surgery commitments, he continued: 'I'm also faced by this pressure of not wanting the consultation to be too long. So there's hesitancy from that point of view, of opening up a new area in a consultation that might very well take another twenty minutes.' He was uncomfortable with the result, as it conflicted with the value he placed on openness. Yet, as he conceded, surgery demands tended to win in the end.

Other doctors were also anxious to prevent matters from getting out of hand, but they viewed the situation less flexibly. They, too, resolved the empathy–detachment question in favour of the latter, principally by observing time-limits and carefully scheduling their workloads. Although GPs were uneasy, the use of these strategies protected them from becoming more involved. Anxieties were minimized. Several GPs commented on the time-consuming nature of such 'feeling work'. Dr Black, for instance, thought:

The problem is that all these things like explaining things, listening, exploring, all take time. If a rush comes you just haven't got it. And I think GPs, unless they've got a very small list, just aren't able to give time. Certainly I've got to see a lot more patients than I've got time to do the way I'd like to see them.

Dr Richards also felt that giving emotional support was difficult for doctors to do well because it took time. In addition, he thought that patients were unwilling to express their concerns about growing helplessness and deterioration to their doctors for fear of having them confirmed, a situation which he would personally find very upsetting. Giving less room for patients to express their distress simplified matters: anxieties were kept at a safe distance. The demands of a busy surgery took precedence. These GPs felt less able to reorder their time. They paced themselves more strictly. Precisely because the use of time involves value judgements, it indicates that other considerations than the ticking of the clock are at stake. GPs regretted being unable to open up the consultation but were resigned to the fact—and perhaps relieved—that 'pressures of work' absolved them from a task which was likely to prove distressing and to heighten their own anxieties about being able to cope.

The tension between the ideal of responding to patients' inner pain and the perceived impracticality of doing so was most vividly illustrated by Dr Quinn. Over the years, he had resolved the question of how far to go by 'not getting too involved'. Exploring patients' troubles had been a luxury:

> You're always trying to make short cuts in general practice because you have to get your day's work done. And you're always thinking of your patients waiting in the waiting-room who've been waiting for an hour. They're waiting at eleven for a ten o'clock appointment and there you are, you're running late and you just have to get patients out of the surgery. Although of course you would like to talk to them much more than that. . . . So have GPs time for counselling patients? They do their best.

In his desire to be fair to all his patients, time was a very real constraint. However, it could be used differently. With experience of his wife's cancer, Dr Quinn wrote to me some time later saying how differently he would approach his work now. His fear of cancer had disappeared and he hoped that he would be able to allay his patients' anxieties. As he explained fear had been a major force behind the detachment he had evolved over the years.

COMMENT

In deciding how far to encourage patients to talk about their troubles, all GPs in the study were engaged in striking a balance between empathy and detachment which was workable for them. However, their conclusions differed, with important implications for communication with their patients. Time—how it was interpreted and used—was critical in determining the balance.

Some doctors felt that they had come to terms with human suffering and had revised their work priorities to allow time and space to respond to its demands. The ability to contain the anxieties which patients' distress might arouse in themselves allowed them to be open to patients' deeper concerns. They felt that this helped patients to cope in their everyday lives. Doctors paced themselves accordingly. Nevertheless, they, too, were affected to some degree by the constraints of surgery pressures. Empathy was qualified.

Other GPs were more detached. The fear of losing control sometimes led them, however regretfully, to opt for a less expansive view of how far to go. There was 'not enough time' for exploring patients' worries. Doctors doubted their ability to control the inner disquiet which opening the discussion to patients might raise in themselves. They preferred not to risk it and allocated less time to the problem of patients seeking to reconcile themselves to their situation.

LISTENING, AND JUST BEING THERE: *'As far as emotional support goes, I think that's quite difficult for doctors to do properly'*

The complementary activity to that of inviting patients to talk about their troubles is listening and responding to what patients say. The ability to listen to, rather than talk at, others is an elusive distinction to clarify, as Jefferys and Sachs (1983) pointed out of some of the GPs they studied. The former is a creative process, requiring an active engagement by the listener. Real listening is hard work. It demands involvement. By contrast, talking at, or the interpretation of listening simply as not talking, are more passive processes which require less commitment.

An important part of listening is just being there—a metaphorical holding of hands. Studies have shown how difficult these tasks are for doctors. Tuckett *et al.* (1985, p. 215) comment: '. . . noticing what patients are thinking and feeling may often increase personal doubt and uncertainty, increase unwanted feelings of emotional involvement, and increase a sense of helplessness.' In managing a chronic illness such as P.D., creative listening and providing a comforting presence are, I believe, vitally important. They indicate that a doctor understands and cares about the patient's human predicament—perhaps the most valuable task a GP can perform for his/her patients.

Listening

The way GPs in the study approached these closely related tasks had important implications for the kind of relationships they established with their P.D. patients. All GPs emphasized the importance of listening. However, their interpretation of this activity varied. Some doctors considered that 'listening as therapy' was a vital part of their professional role. They made room for any uncertainty this might arouse, having learnt to deal with it positively and openly. They shared patients' struggles to cope.

Dr Perlmann and Dr Threadgold illustrated the dynamic nature of the listening process. 'I think one empathizes and one reflects and one sympathizes with patients' needs and emotions, and tries to help the patient understand their own feelings in a sort of reflective way' (Dr Perlmann). Dr Threadgold amplified this:

> Quite a lot of the process is involved in just being a sponge to *listen* and hear what someone's worries are. . . . And I may very well just share their distress with them. I may very well put back in various things. I may put back an understanding of their distress in terms of 'That is perfectly reasonable because anyone in your situation would feel like that'. 'I guess that's actually worse for you because of what happened to your Granny last year.' . . . I may be helping them to understand a bit why they're distressed. . . . I'm saying 'It's your problem, you've got to cope with it', but I'm also saying 'I'll help you cope with it'.

While all GPs in the study grappled with the task of striking a workable balance between empathy and detachment, some doctors, able to give more room for manoeuvre than others, resolved the question in favour of openness. They enjoyed the involvement which listening allowed. They were receptive to—and expected—'lots of emotional reactions' (Dr Young). Patients were encouraged to express their troubles to ease the job of coming to terms with the illness. Listening in this way did not leave GPs feeling inadequate or helpless.

Creative listening was also a passport to understanding what the illness experience meant for patients' lives. Dr Ellis thought that:

> A lot of this looking after chronic illness has to do with how you would feel in that situation. I suppose that's what medicine is, trying to put yourself in someone else's position. How *do* you cope with a stiff hip? Inside you want to be running for the bus or you want to dash upstairs to get your spectacles. You can't do it. If you as a doctor can't appreciate how frustrating that must be, in other words if you only see that osteoarthritic hip, then you're doomed to a lousy doctor–patient relationship.

She understood the difficult task of translating clinical knowledge of the condition into an understanding of what this meant for patients' lives. Moreover, she needed this understanding to be able to respond effectively and sensitively. There was room for the person behind the patient to emerge.

Dr Leadbrough also found the development of understanding one of the most rewarding parts of her work and confessed that she would be very bored without it. Nevertheless, as other GPs in the study who had a commitment to openness found, she, too, had her limits. In stressful situations where she felt in danger of being overwhelmed, she thought 'There's always professionalism to fall back on. You can't always be empathizing to the *n*th degree.' She was careful to take things on 'in small packages' and not to overload herself with 'too many distressing cases at once'.

It was apparent that other doctors had rather different ideas about listening from those of the GPs just described. While Dr Victor rarely felt threatened by anxiety, it emerged that his approach emphasized actively guiding and advising patients. He said: 'I think I have a reputation for being not exactly a lazy doctor, but part of the time I just talk to them. . . . I spend much more time talking to patients and asking about their symptoms.' Interpreting the task of listening in this way allowed him to distance himself from the possibility of being overwhelmed by patients' distress.

Dr Naughton illustrated a further distinction between talking and 'being company'. Consistent with his views on explaining what to expect, he relied more on patients to take the initiative:

> Yes I certainly think I've got time to talk about problems, particularly if the patient brings them up. What I don't necessarily see myself as having the time to do is to sit down and be company . . . loneliness is one of the biggest problems and when I started here I made the mistake, with the best of intentions, of trying to treat loneliness by myself. And one simply can't do it and do all these other things as well. . . . Having said that, I do hope I don't reject a response by a patient.

His practice had previously been very elderly-oriented. He had recently rescheduled his work to include preventive services such as screening for rubella and hypertension. This meant sacrificing some of the listening which had been a high priority before. He regretted the shift that this entailed in the balance between empathy and detachment, but felt that it was more appropriate to modern practice.

Listening seemed to be a passive process for Dr Wilkinson, to be 'got through' rather than creatively used as providing insights into the ways patients came to grips with suffering. Listening was interpreted as not talking or interrupting. Consistent with his wish 'not to get too involved with anyone', he described his response to patients' distress: 'You've just got to sit and wait and chat through it until it's all finished. You normally get tears in the surgery only when they haven't been able to have floods of tears somewhere else. So I sit there and wait until it's all over and carry on then.' Like other GPs in the study, he was concerned with 'watching the limits, otherwise you'll end up exhausting yourself'. He kept a firm grip on how far to go, preferring to give less priority to active listening. The adoption of a more closed approach enabled anxieties to be kept at bay and prevented him from feeling overwhelmed.

Finally, Dr Quinn illustrated most vividly the difficulties which coping with the social and emotional crises of his chronically sick patients raised. Listening was closely rationed, with an eye on the clock. He could not risk losing control or exposing his own fears and anxieties which creative listening might activate. He said: 'Certainly you spend all the time you can with them, listening. I think the great thing is to listen to patients. And put in the odd word here and there. But again it's a question of time. You only have five minutes per patient. We do our best. It's all very difficult.' The tension between trying to reconcile the task of coping efficiently with a given volume of work with a view of himself as a caring, compassionate doctor had taken on a new dimension with his wife's illness. He explained further:

> Well you should never get involved with one's patients because there are so many diseases that you soon find you aren't working efficiently if you get involved with all your patients. You have to keep a distance. That's where it comes in, you see. When it's your family you have to get involved. That's the difference. . . . I think doctors see things from a different point of view from the lay public. It's really a question of being involved, I think personally, as with my wife's cancer. . . . You see you're talking from one side of the fence to the other side of the fence.

Throughout his working life he had adopted a fairly closed approach to his patients' distress. The contrast between his views on his work as a GP and the personal experience of being cast with his wife into the sick role poignantly highlighted the gap between doctor and patient, between professional knowledge and subjective experience of managing the fears cancer raised.

These GPs evidently expected patients to cope with these potentially distressing areas of the P.D. experience outside the confines of the surgery. The task of translating knowledge into understanding—and thus bridging the gap between knowledge and experience—was too complex and threatening. These GPs felt that it was beyond the scope of their work. Experience with, and experience of, are on different conceptual levels. Doctors felt more comfortable confining their work to the former activity.

Just Being There

A crucial part of listening is the ability to be comfortable with just being beside the patient, not necessarily contributing anything specifically medical to the encounter. Dr Young explained:

> You can alleviate suffering very often just by being there yourself, and I think it's important to recognize that as an important thing to do. . . . I think that's the important function of a doctor, just to alleviate suffering. I know it sounds trite. . . . I don't know whether it comes to you as you get older. I'm getting better at it. I get less frustrated now with people who actually don't ever get any better. I think all you can really offer is time for people to come and talk to you about things.

It took time and sometimes involved confronting painful difficulties of their own for doctors to be comfortable with this aspect of general practice. Dr Young had had what she described as 'a serious depressive illness' as a result of the strain involved in trying to take on too much. She paced herself more cautiously, without, however, sacrificing her openness to patients' needs.

These GPs adopted quite elaborate strategies to enable them to survive. Dr Richards and Dr Young emphasized the liberating effect that 'being honest' with patients had on their ability to deal with both their own and their patients' anxieties. They also relied on support from their colleagues or counselling groups to help to sort out their priorities and come to terms with their own physical and personal limitations—as well as with the limitations of medicine itself. The presence of supportive colleagues made a great difference to the lives of Dr Clements and Dr Ellis—in sharp contrast to Dr Perlmann and Dr Wilkinson, who worked single-handed. Moreover, Dr Ellis was not afraid to show her own feelings to her patients:

> I think talking to other people of like minds helps. We've got a practice where we can go and say to one another 'I'm going to kick the cat if you don't talk to me or listen to what I've just had to go through'. And I think I'd find it very difficult if I didn't have that sort of professional relationship in my practice. . . . I cry a lot. I don't cry sort of 'sob, sob, sob', but I find I cry with people a lot. If they feel sad and I feel sad it sort of comes out. I used to think it was embarrassing to the patients. I started to cover it up, but there's no point.

The open acknowledgement of her own sympathy with her patients' plight enabled her to respond better. She felt it also helped patients to adjust to the often tragic dimensions of life with P.D. The process of sharing fears and sadness—grieving openly with patients—was a way of healing. Listening and just being with patients were fundamental to that task.

Four doctors had arranged their practices so that more emphasis could be given to this aspect of their work. They created time and space for sharing patients' troubles. Dr Miller had been initially attracted to neurology because of the time she was able to devote to individual patients. Commenting on her work as a GP, she said: 'I think brushing over things is fairly typical of general practice with the six-minute consultation. We in our practice have ten minutes and have half-an-hour about every hour so that we could be spending an average of fifteen minutes with every patient.' Because she considered that sharing distress with patients was an important part of general practice, time was apportioned accordingly. Indeed, available time was managed somewhat differently.

Other GPs, anxious to contain what they took on, often felt awkward with the 'non-activity' which just being there implied. Doctors were uncomfortable dealing with P.D. patients and their families where conventional medical intervention was no longer appropriate. They felt intensely vulnerable. Again there was often no yardstick by which to judge the value of what they were doing. Dr Richards has already described the discomfort he felt with the limitations of the treatment. He went on: 'I think having someone to talk to does help. But I always feel I should *do* something with the problem they've produced, but I suppose that isn't always the case.'

Dr Fleming had similar difficulties. In addition, his comment reflects the discomfort raised by the age difference between many GPs in the study and the typically older P.D. patient. As discussed earlier, empathy with the elderly is difficult for the young to achieve at the best of times. It means appreciating 'this could be me in twenty years' time'. Trying to empathize with the elderly chronic sick was doubly hard. Dr Fleming explained:

> I think that a large part of one's pastoral care role is going to see the patient and maintaining that contact. And I think it can be something very difficult to do as a young GP. I think it's something that takes time to be comfortable with, that is going into someone's house, sitting down, passing the time of day with them, *not* doing anything at all in a medical sense. . . . Whether you do anything in a medical sense or not, that is a very important role I think.

While providing a comforting presence was seen as a vital part of general practice, these GPs also felt anxious. Although Dr Ogilvie said that he 'rarely felt completely helpless' and Dr Richards thought that 'by sharing a patient's helplessness with them it actually makes the relationship more straightforward', many felt inadequate at being unable tangibly to alleviate suffering. It was difficult for doctors to feel that they were being effective in a straightforward way. Dr Black candidly acknowledged the profound anxieties that responding openly to patients' distress raised. He spoke for many GPs in the study: 'I think it's one of the most difficult things to do. In one way one rather dreads it. In one way you can do so little to help. I mean you can try, but I think my reaction's one of inadequacy when faced with this sort of problem.' The task of sharing patients' pain was potentially distressing. He preferred to avoid such a situation, where possible.

The absence of any clear-cut professional guidelines in these uncharted areas of work increased uncertainty. This was compounded by the lack of positive indication that 'non-activity' directly benefited patients. Dr Black wanted to see some definite 'pay-off' before listening to or being beside patients could be taken as a worth-while investment of time. While he felt 'very good' if a patient told him directly how helpful listening had been, he was at a loss to know whether his services had been of use when this confirmation was absent. The tasks of listening and support do not readily lend themselves to the visible evaluation provided by, for example, a patient's response to medication.

Those GPs in the study who recognized the importance of these activities but felt diffident about their ability to cope were perhaps most vulnerable to feelings of unease. They recognized that dealing with chronic illness needed a different, less dispassionate approach to that of acute conditions, but often found the anxieties this approach raised difficult to handle. They opted for greater professional detachment, a position with which more experienced doctors, such as Dr Victor and Dr Dandridge, felt more comfortable.

SUMMARY AND COMMENT

The evidence has shown the difficulties many GPs found in exploring patients' deeper worries and in listening or providing a reassuring presence. All GPs wanted to keep uncertainty at a manageable level, but the definition of what was manageable varied. Different GPs were able to handle differing amounts of involvement with their patients' distress. Some GPs were receptive to patients who wanted to grieve openly. Others were less so. Their patients evidently had to look elsewhere for such support.

Some doctors preferred to commit themselves more actively to tackling patients' human concerns. They were confident that this was a vital part of general practice. They evolved particular ways of managing potential anxieties: by a flexible approach to time, by the use of pacing strategies and by reliance on the support of colleagues or counselling groups. They felt that they had come to terms with their own feelings about human suffering so that involvement, within limits, was less of a strain. Some understanding of the experience of chronic illness accompanied clinical knowledge of the condition. The disparity between knowledge and experience was, in some measure, bridged.

Other doctors adopted a more closed approach to what they were prepared to take on. Opening up the consultation was too risky. GPs recognized instinctively that, once started on that slippery slope, there could be no stopping; they would either end up as Mother Theresas or cease functioning altogether. They resolved the situation by rationing time more strictly and by giving their patients less room for manoeuvre. Doctors did not necessarily want to make the leap from knowledge of P.D. as a clinical entity to understanding the P.D. experience. However, some GPs were not always comfortable with this position, yet feared the alternatives.

GPs often keenly felt the lack of feedback that such intervention helped their patients. They found the mask-like face and speech difficulties of some P.D. patients disconcerting. Cues were often missing and doctors were uncertain as to whether their services were of value.

Moreover, doctors often felt the task of sustaining the quality of care for their P.D. patients over a long time-span to be stressful. They appreciated that medicine had, in a sense, failed the chronically ill. As medical practitioners, it was difficult not to take this failure personally.

This is not to underestimate the difficulties GPs faced. Routinely they had to confront human suffering and emerge unscathed at the end of the day. Doctors were understandably reluctant to be drawn into spending time exploring areas which were potentially fraught with anxiety. They were in unknown territory. All they had for guidance were their own personal inclinations and a variable understanding of their own strengths and limitations.

It is important to emphasize that although this was a more stressful area of work than that of explanation-giving or managing treatment (and was acknowledged as such), GPs were not so plagued by doubts that they were unable to make any decisions. As shown, they had developed routines to handle uncertainty. They did their very best.

Dr Quinn raised an important issue: Is the GP the most appropriate person to take on such a task? The GP is saddled with a difficult problem: he/she is a specialist in *general* practice. There are many competing demands on his/her time and attention, and skills in empathy are not easy to acquire. Yet a GP is often the first port of call for patients. A sensitive response at that critical time may make or mar future relations. *Caritas* surely implies having an awareness of patients' inner disquiet and some understanding of what is likely to be happening. Attending to patients' innermost feelings is just as important as handling strictly medical matters. The following chapter will show how vital such sensitivity is for patients.

7

Controlling the Uncontrollable: Making Sense of Living with P.D.

INTRODUCTION

As we have seen in Chapters 3 and 5, patients sought to reduce uncertainty by controlling the pace of assimilating what to expect of the illness, and by developing some expertise in handling the medication. Crucially, patients also tried to control the uncertainties—and the inner disquiet which accompanied them—of the illness experience itself, in ways very different from those described by the GPs in the previous chapter. Moreover, as argued previously, the uncertainties *themselves* were different. Again these differences had important implications for the patient–GP relationship.

Patients in the study were as much concerned to give meaning to the broader issues of having P.D. as to address questions of cause. The problem was less one of 'why have I got Parkinson's now?' than 'what am I to make of life now that this has happened?' (Williams and Wood, 1986). This meant dealing with basic questions about the meaning or meaninglessness of patients' new lives. As chronic illness is lived and experienced mostly in the home rather than in the GP's surgery, it is to these experiences that I now turn.

This chapter explores some of the fears and anxieties having P.D. held for patients: fears of the wheelchair and attendant loss of independence, of becoming what is often disagreeably termed a 'vegetable', of losing mental faculties, and of helplessness in a culture which values independence and self-reliance. It then briefly explores the main strategies patients used to make sense of these fears—patients wanted to live as normally as possible and many fought hard to do so—and considers how the scope for controlling uncertainty became increasingly precarious as the illness progressed. The chapter concludes by exploring how far patients felt their GPs helped them in these tasks and, indeed, how far they felt it was appropriate for their GPs to do so.

IDENTITY UNDER THREAT: *'I suppose it makes me feel geriatric really'*

Patients were most distressed by the prospect of dependence and by intense feelings of loss. The fear of becoming a burden was particularly acute (see Bury, 1982; Charmaz, 1983; Locker, 1983). Both fear of, and frustration with, helplessness affected patients in the study. The protracted nature of P.D. made the threat of losing control of one's body particularly hard to bear. Mr Canning reflected:

MR CANNING: Long-term illness has always been a dread of mine. My neighbour dropped down dead whilst he was putting the kettle on. . . . In the long run what a way to go while you're making a cup of tea for yourself!
R.P.: What are the things about it you find so fearful?
MR CANNING: I suppose living like a cabbage for so long.

References to 'being a vegetable' or 'being a cabbage', with their associated images of helplessness and loss of physical and mental control, were frequently made by patients.

When anticipation became actuality, patients were often intensely frustrated. Mrs Unwin told me how her husband banged his stick on the floor in rage at his impotence. Mr Unwin remarked that although he had 'got used to it now, having to be helped', it was still hard '. . . having to ask people to come and help you, and waiting for 'em to come and help. You've got nothing to give in place of it.' Mrs Unwin said: 'It's having to rely on other people.' The lack of 'exchange currency' with which to reciprocate—often experienced by the dependent elderly (Dowd, 1975)—was particularly galling. Patients felt that they had little to offer of comparable value. Relationships with others were uncomfortably off-balance.

Fear of dependence often focused on the wheelchair. It marked a point of no return. My Vernon, although agreeing that this was not how things should be, nevertheless felt: 'It represents a sort of rejection in a way by society. Not a rejection, but an acknowledgement of failure.' For Mr Dempsey it represented total defeat: 'The last thing I want is a wheelchair. I don't want my children have to finish up putting me in the bath and getting me out of the bath and feeding me. . . . Once I'm immobile totally there's nothing left. You might as well kill yourself. I'd rather die than that.' The wheelchair was a symbolic staging post. It marked a point in time when patients defined themselves as dependent and therefore undesirably different, not only from others, but also from a former part of themselves.

Fear of or frustration with having to rely on others for help with the most basic bodily functions of daily life were closely linked to feelings of loss. These were expressed both generally and specifically in terms of the loss of previously valued capacities, skills and activities. Some patients were particularly affected when they could no longer perform physical tasks which they had previously taken for granted. Mrs Franklin, for example, felt:

> That's the worst thing, the lack of grace. I used to have a friend who said to me that I was deft. I've lost that deftness and I don't like it. I come out of the bank with money, a purse, handbag and umbrella and I don't *know* how to put them away. I've got to *think* which hand to move first. I resent being ungraceful and clumsy.

Patients had to accept a new Identikit which was often at odds with the way they had previously defined themselves. Mr Canning voiced the feelings of several patients who had been proud of their physical fitness prior to the illness: 'You see I've never been unable to do anything I wanted to. Physically there's been no question. If I wanted to take up something I would do it. I can't now.'

Patients also grieved at the loss of particular abilities and activities. Several patients commented on the deterioration in mental agility and the ability to communicate effectively. Mr Jenson, for example, said: 'I've lost the ability to do all sorts of things. Technically I'm not as quick-witted as I was. If I was involved in an argument or debate I miss out. . . . In middle management one expects to be able to do this kind of thing.' Handicap prevented patients from pursuing valued activities which had given them a sense of who they were. Such losses represented an assault on self-hood. Vital pieces of the self were being eroded, leaving patients bereft, their very identities in question.

Feelings of loss also found expression in increasing social isolation (Charmaz, 1983; Cobb and Hamera, 1986). Several patients described how the illness had restricted their social lives. Mrs York reflected:

> Another thing which is rather frightening and horrible is that as the thing progresses, friends and acquaintances seem to vanish because they don't know how to cope. So they don't come easily any more because they don't know what to say and what to do. And lots of people say they are praying for me and I say 'Well, thank you very much', and lots of people ring me up but hardly ever say 'How's your husband?' I think they're scared.

As a devalued status, chronic illness made normal contact with others difficult. Social isolation was also circular. Leading a restricted life caused withdrawal from others, which in turn increased social isolation. Mrs York found herself doubly isolated. With her husband's virtual inability to speak, she was imprisoned in a world of silence.

Patients' marriages also came under strain. The illness of one partner often meant the loss of privacy, the inability to go out in case of accident and the reversal of long-valued roles. Frequent mood changes were also disturbing, as Mrs Mitchell found of her husband:

MRS MITCHELL: Since he's had Parkinson's, he's gone very moody, very very moody. . . . We didn't know what a row was before he had Parkinson's. You know

what I mean when I say a row. But now we have thundering good rows.
MR MITCHELL: I wouldn't say it's a good thing. It's made life unbearable.
MRS MITCHELL: It's damaged our marriage. That's what he's trying to say.

Other spouses felt trapped in a relationship that resembled less a marriage
and more a nurse–patient relationship. As most patients were retired, the
loss of social contacts and strained marital relationships were correspondingly harder to bear.

IN SEARCH OF CONTROL: *'I think the one most important thing to me at
the moment is controlling the illness I've got. That's the thing that takes most
of my time up'*

Patients could not, and did not, remain passive in the face of such
difficulties. Almost all, whatever their degree of disability, made strenuous
efforts to maintain life as normally as possible, a pattern characteristic of
other chronically ill patients (Strauss and Glaser, 1975; Pearlin and
Schooler, 1978; Anderson and Bury, 1988). Again managing uncertainty
tended to reflect a broader outlook on life's trials and tribulations as much
as the development of specific techniques to be mastered in response to the
particular difficulties of P.D. Strategies which were helpful in one life
situation were adapted or modified to meet this new situation.

The most common device used was that of fighting the fears and
forebodings which the illness raised. Patients strove to preserve as much of
their normal selves as possible. The interweaving of both philosophical and
practical responses was illustrated by the following, fairly typical, remarks
of Mr Vernon and Mrs Quentin. They had developed a positive, almost
combative, approach to living with P.D. Mr Vernon described how he and
his wife viewed the situation:

> We both feel that this is something that has got to be lived with, that one should
> fight as hard as possible to retain independence of movement and one should do
> the things one enjoys doing. . . . I think the best thing to do is to fight to retain
> mobility and energy. One has to continue to drive and continue to walk, and
> that's my basic philosophy.

Mrs Quentin emphasized the more practical response she had developed,
which nonetheless also reflected her outlook on life. She exploited her
residual physical capacities to the utmost to be in charge.

> I do work on things. I do the exercises. And I do the walks. They taught me to
> march and of course we've got lots of nice corridors here [sheltered housing].
> When I go to empty my rubbish I march there and march back. I think that's
> helped with my walking because there's a fear of taking those little steps that I
> see some people doing. I do think it helps if you march along. . . . I have a terror
> of this shuffling people do.

Fighting strategies which were part and parcel of making sense of being a P.D. patient took time, effort and ingenuity, so that they became a form of 'hidden work' (Wadel, 1979)—rarely acknowledged as such by either health professionals or patients themselves. The routines patients developed were geared towards a specific result (or product): holding the negative feelings in check to achieve a measure of control over the inner terrors the illness raised in them.

Patients also felt that over time they came to accept the illness, without necessarily giving in to it. Miss Norton's friend, who later became her husband, said of her: 'Parkinson's is one of those accepted things. She keeps it more or less in the background. It hasn't taken over. She's not sitting thinking about it all day and every day. She's accepted it. She knows it can't be remedied.' However, it would be a mistake to consider such acceptance as a form of capitulation. As we have seen earlier, those patients who felt that they 'accepted' the situation were accepting the fact of having P.D. rather than accepting the various personal and social consequences of the illness. Nevertheless, the relationship between fighting and acceptance was complex. Mr Grenville illustrated the tension between the two, and the partial resolution he had made:

> On the one hand you've got Fate to accept, and yet you've got these human attributes with which to fight and resist, as if you've got self-determination. Because the logical consequence of belief and acceptance of Fate is that you don't fight and resist, so this is the big conflict . . . one should accept it [Fate] at one level but fight it and resist it on another.

Acceptance of the irrevocability of the illness—that it had happened to them—did not mean that patients ceased grappling with its consequences; rather the contrary. If fears were to be controlled, recipes for making sense of life with P.D. had to be developed.

Moreover, patients defined their physical disabilities in ways which allowed them to preserve a sense of who they were. Thus, Miss Norton, for example, was able to refer to herself as only 'mildly handicapped', even though she was virtually unable to speak. The illness experience was more than just a cluster of physical symptoms. It held particular meanings for patients. If they were to survive, these had to be woven into the fabric of patients' lives in a way that confirmed their integrity.

Two sub-strategies were important in helping patients maintain a sense of control: the use of referents and the restructuring of time perspectives.

(1) The use of referents, both negative and positive, was common. The sight of other P.D. patients much worse than themselves allowed some patients to see themselves as possible exceptions to the rule. They could locate their own position on an imagined scale of handicap with more equanimity when faced with the contrast. Both Mr and Mrs Jenson found

the Parkinson's Disease Society Branch meetings helpful in this respect:

> MR JENSON: There's a range of people there and I'm worse than some and better than others.
> R.P.: So you make comparisons?
> MR JENSON: Oh *yes*!
> MRS JENSON: In my mind whenever things have seemed down I think to myself 'that feller's worse than J!'

Patients could distance themselves from the image when they were less obviously handicapped themselves. Mr Jenson was different. Again this should not be interpreted pejoratively as denial. Distancing was an essential survival device. Patients felt they were still in charge of the impact of the illness on them.

On the other hand, positive referents gave patients hope. They provided a model patients could emulate. Mrs Franklin mused:

> Katherine Hepburn, she's had Parkinson's a long time. . . . She has, I think, a similar type of Parkinson's, a bit like me. She's obviously got a bit worse but not much. And she's another one who's decided right at the beginning she's going to get on with her career and to hell with it. And she's got on top of it. I didn't at the beginning but I think I did after a while.

If one person could make a success of life with the illness, so could others.

Thus, the use of referents either helped patients to distance themselves as different, allowing them to construct an optimistic view of their own condition by contrast, or provided them with models with whom to identify.

(2) Patients also restructured their time perspectives as a means of controlling uncertainty. With the onset of P.D., the future dimension tended to collapse. It could no longer be taken for granted that patients had a future in the way others conceive of life as moving smoothly through a past, a present and a future. Most patients, particularly those more seriously handicapped, commented on this, saying 'I live from day to day', or 'I take one day at a time', or 'I don't plan too far into the future'. They focused on the present. The future was virtually eliminated as a threat too anxiety-provoking to contemplate. Even for the mildly handicapped, temporal horizons had shrunk. Miss Evans said:

> You can't think about the future, you've got to think about the present. I can't plan anything. I just take each day as it comes. It doesn't mean I don't make plans for going out and that sort of thing, but I don't make plans for how I'm going to live my life because I don't think you can when you've got a disease which is progressive. It might be a bit to do with the fact that you're afraid of thinking about the future.

Patients were intent on getting as much out of life now as possible, even though parts of the present had to be written off as 'dead time', as Mr

Dempsey's experience of juggling the medication has shown. He described his approach:

> I'm going to get as much fun out of today as I can and worry about tomorrow tomorrow. I'm not going to worry myself stiff so's I don't go out. Putting it bluntly I couldn't be a miserable bugger. You don't want to live that way do you? You think life's a hope. You hope that it doesn't happen and ignore it if you can.

It was an outlook adopted well before the onset of P.D. Referring to his attitude to money, he had remarked earlier: 'You don't want to be the richest person in the graveyard do you.' His philosophy was as much a recipe for accomplishing life as a carefully measured response to the uncertainties of P.D.

At the same time, the past was disconnected from the present. It was irretrievable. Patients found that they were able to erase memories of previous experience of life without P.D. Mrs Franklin mused: 'I can't remember what it was like before I had it. I can remember lists of things that I did and can't do now, but I can't actually remember what it was like *doing* them.' Freedom of movement seemed to belong to another world. On one level this was a serious loss. On another, fading memory helped reduce the pain which accompanied that 'loss of self' which is fundamental to the experience of chronic illness (Charmaz, 1983). The human capacity to forget was a blessing. It helped patients to survive. Hazan's (1980) study of residents at a Centre for the Elderly has referred to the 'cognitive obliteration' of past and future as a means of being in charge. Patients managed P.D. in very similar ways: they blotted out memories of the past and refused to anticipate the future. Indeed, as P.D. is typically an illness of later years, it placed additional pressures on patients to restructure their ideas on time. Focus on the present was all-important.

MAKING A PACT WITH P.D.: *'I know you learn by experience, but whether you can be absolutely in control . . .'*

As the illness developed, it became increasingly difficult to rely on these controlling devices. Anxiety was rekindled as new symptoms developed. Once again the question of what living with P.D. meant moved to the forefront of patients' attention. They often recognized that control could not be sustained at length. For varying parts of a day or a week, the illness took over. Mr Vernon noted: 'I would qualify that [idea of control] by adding that the control function gets harder as you go along. You are constantly having to readjust your control mechanisms to a worse level of disability.' As patients wove in and out of control, routines had to be continuously rethought. Sometimes patients negotiated a compromise. Mrs Franklin conceded: 'It can have five minutes of my time but no more!' Over time, however, the bargain became more elastic, as the illness occupied increasing areas of life. Mr Irving was more seriously handicapped. He commented:

> I can see the time coming when it's going to be less and less possible to do the kind of living I want. . . . My idea is to do everything that I can do and at some stage, I suppose, say 'Well, look, enough is enough'. There was a man in hospital with me. I wouldn't have lived like that because he was a cabbage. He *was* an intelligent man.

With the death of his wife and his subsequent transfer to residential care, he was increasingly aware of life closing in around him. His ability to 'put on a show' for visitors became erratic and often could not be sustained during a visit. A surprise lunch party he gave in honour of this manuscript was curtailed by his withdrawal into frozen immobility. Nevertheless, he had recaptured, for a brief interlude, something of his former self.

Similarly, Mrs Quentin's increasingly debilitating muscle spasms taxed her resources to the limit. Their unpredictability made family life, which was dear to her, difficult to maintain. The loss of control and its accompanying anxiety distressed her: 'These spasms don't have a pattern. If they did you could weave your life around them. But they strike for no reason at all.' However, when she was free from pain, she expended every effort to put visitors at ease and ensure that her grandchildren were not exposed to her own distress. Strategies had to be adapted and readapted to changing circumstances, but they were not totally abandoned. Patients still struggled to engage with the world.

COMMENT

Patients had to manage fears of dependency and the sense of loss which distressed them if they were to carry on. The development of strategies was thus vitally important in gaining a purchase on the inner forebodings which living with P.D. raised.

Patients sought to preserve their identity in the face of physical changes to their bodies. If this meant devoting three times as much energy to accomplishing tasks which they had previously taken for granted, or forfeiting parts of the day and even the future itself, such compromises enabled patients to survive with their self-respect relatively intact. This is a process in which we are all engaged over our life-course, but one which is particularly poignant for people with P.D.

These routines complemented the other steps, described earlier, which patients took to manage information and develop know-how in handling the medication. They constituted a body of expertise in controlling the uncontrollable. Ironically, perhaps, they represented denial of the one certainty patients did have: that the illness would not get better and would, in all probability, get worse.

The crucial questions to which I shall now turn were: How did patients feel their GPs responded to these concerns? What role, if any, did they play in these vital areas of patients' lives? Were the fears and anxieties which haunted patients communicated to their GPs and, if so, how?

HOW MUCH CAN THE GP OFFER?

The absence or presence of a caring GP in this vital area of patient concern made a great difference to the way patients were able to manage. For the majority of patients in the study (ten), their GP was of little significance. For the others, a supportive GP helped to make the illness experience more bearable.

A Marginal Figure

'I've never had any support from him, so I cope myself'
Three patients felt that their GPs neither were interested in nor cared about the concerns just discussed. Both Mr and Mrs Jenson and Mr and Mrs Mitchell had approached their GP for help. Mr and Mrs Jenson described one encounter:

MR JENSON: I went to him with depression once.
R.P.: How did that go?
MRS JENSON: Another pill.
MR JENSON: He says 'How are you doing?' and I tell him and there's very little reaction.
R.P.: What do you think you're looking for that's missing?
MR JENSON: Well I'm looking for relief of my suffering but I don't get it.
R.P.: I wonder what would relieve it?
MR JENSON: Probably the sort of thing we're doing right now. Discussing it!

The apparent invitation to explore Mr Jenson's feelings was not pursued. His GP responded to his depression at a clinical, rather than at a human, level.

Further, it was difficult to put complex feelings into words. Standard phrases which patients hoped would elicit a warm response fell on deaf ears as Mr Mitchell found when he consulted his GP feeling 'edgy and moody':

MR MITCHELL: He says 'Well carry on with the tablets and I'll see you in a month's time'.
MRS MITCHELL: When M. said he'd got stress the doctor just laughed.
R.P.: What kind of a laugh was that?
MRS MITCHELL: 'Ah-ha [snorts], Oh, piffle, I-can't-be-bothered' kind of a laugh.

These patients translated their concerns into what they felt was an appropriate vocabulary with which to consult doctors. However, they were profoundly distressed by the lack of affective response to their unspoken needs. Neither couple felt that their GPs were addressing the meanings which 'being depressed' held for them. Their GPs were not really listening. Patients felt rebuffed; their inner distress was heightened. This is not to suggest that there is always an underlying reason for depression. It may well be a perfectly normal biological accompaniment of the disease. But these were the concerns likely to be troubling patients.

Anxiety was compounded when patients found themselves being sent back and forth between GP and consultant in their quest for someone who might address their needs. After the death of his wife, Mr Dempsey developed severe chest pains similar to those of his late wife. His GP sent him to see the neurologist who was treating his P.D., who in turn referred him straight back to his GP, saying: '"Me? I'm not a GP. I don't do that sort of business anyway. . . . It's no good seeing me. I don't know nothing about things like that. Best thing you can do is to go down to your GP tomorrow. I'll write a letter anyway, but tell him it's no good your coming up here".' Eventually Mr Dempsey was referred to his local hospital, where he was 'talked out of it'. His GP's initial failure to attend to his distress had important consequences for any future patient–GP relationship. He considered it a 'waste of time' visiting the surgery: 'I think probably in my mind the GP can't do much for me so I don't bother.' Anxiety was often high. The prospect of future support for these patients seemed bleak. They did not know where to turn.

Several patients felt either that their GP could not be expected to help them make sense of living with P.D. or that it was inappropriate to consult their GP on such a matter. Some patients thought that the present organization of general practice made attention to this impossible. Mrs Franklin said: 'I can't imagine that any of them would have the time or the inclination to do this. Their role is to deal with the biochemical problem and I think the time has gone when the GP can deal with emotional problems.' She contrasted this with 'the old days', when GPs knew their patients' families and, like members of the Church, she thought, would be expected to help. And Mr Vernon, although liking his GP, considered:

> I think I come round to this theory that you've got to treat the whole person. This requires much more sensitivity, intelligence and skill than is displayed at the moment. . . . When it comes to a complex thing like Parkinson's, ideally the GP should think about the family situation, the person's psychological drive and how these might be contributing to making the disease better or worse. . . . But one has to accept that the GP hasn't the time really to see the patient in the way I'm suggesting.

Modern GPs were not expected—nor had they the time—to fulfil a pastoral care role. However, a circular process was in operation here. If doctors were not expected to help in this way, patients would be unlikely to ask for support. In turn, there would be less incentive for doctors to develop appropriate skills. This chicken-and-egg situation made the very changes patients wanted more difficult to achieve, as Roberts (1985) has also noted.

These expectations were closely linked to the feeling expressed by many patients that it was impossible for anyone to understand what having P.D. was like if they had not experienced it themselves. Patients felt that their doctors could not take the half-way step from clinical experience *with* the condition to understanding the nature *of* the experience.

Other patients felt that their GP was not an appropriate person to help with these deeper concerns. The age difference and perceived lack of experience of life were significant in Mr Canning's decision not to approach his GP with depression:

> I wouldn't want to go to him if I was feeling depressed. He's what you might call at the younger end of the GP range and I think I've probably seen more of life than he has. I'm not insulting him but I don't think he has anything to contribute to what I could actually say myself. . . . I wouldn't talk to him about these things because I don't think he's got as much experience as I have. As headmaster I had parents come to me talking about all sorts of things and I have built up a father confessor image. This happens in a headmaster's study, particularly in a poor area, so they'll actually tell you more about themselves than they would to their GP. Now this GP is a lot less experienced than I am, therefore I wouldn't mention things. . . . I don't know whether he's seen the other half of the world, you see.

Again patients did not expect GPs to show the necessary depth of understanding. The lack of experience of poverty and the perceived immaturity of many younger doctors were also important in determining other patients' responses. Mr Grenville felt that he did not need such support from his GP, and Mr Irving commented: 'The doctor plays no part in it at all.' Significantly, he felt unable to discuss the one subject that was increasingly preoccupying him—that of euthanasia—with either GP or consultant. Patients had to turn elsewhere with their despair.

The Person Behind the Patient

'It's necessary with diseases like Parkinson's that you've got doctors who understand you as a person'
By contrast, four patients in the study felt that their GPs were a source of comfort and reassurance, and gave them strength to cope with the fears raised by the illness. These patients felt that they could share their distress with their GPs. Even though patients sometimes had long periods when they rarely saw their GP and considered that they had to be 'ill' to justify an approach, all felt safe. Their GPs were available, and support—whether

implicit or explicit—was forthcoming. Mrs Unwin, for example, said: 'You don't want to go bothering him with those kinds of things [emotional problems]. Just if there's anything wrong.... But he's always said "If you're worried you've only to phone".' Concerns were often so personal that they were not articulated as such. Again it seemed that patients used a different vocabulary when talking with their GPs from that used in describing their fears to a researcher. Nevertheless, Mrs Unwin felt that the mere presence of the GP—just being there—allayed anxiety:

MR UNWIN: It's him himself, isn't it. He's more of a friend.
MRS UNWIN: It's the doctor himself. The doctor's weighing him up all the time. He notices everything.

The couple not only valued the care and befriending their GP had given over the years, but also felt secure in the knowledge that he was keeping a careful eye on things and understood, as far as it was possible for another person to do so, what they were going through.

Sensitivity to the little nuances which make for a caring human relationship mattered to patients as much as did attention to the wider issues. Mrs Quentin recalled: 'When I've gone for prescriptions and it's been icy on the road he always sends a message "Be careful how you go". So you see those little things give you faith in your doctor. It's very important. And when he's talking to you you feel that he cares.' Miss Evans felt that her GP showed similar sensitivity: 'I suppose there is a bond really. I feel he understands perfectly how I feel. I know when I go in he's going to understand what I say.... I don't feel that he doesn't understand the illness or that he hasn't got any sympathy with it.' Confidence in her GP's experience of P.D. was integral to the respect and affection she felt for him. She also felt that he appreciated her 'as a whole person', not just a disease entity—an approach which she considered to be particularly important in managing long-term chronic illnesses. Her GP's interest extended to her hobbies—painting, the flower arrangements she did for the local church—and to her religious faith. He respected concerns which were important to her. The idea of managing P.D. without his help horrified her—a sentiment echoed by Miss Norton, who had become very close to her previous GP. Significantly, she was distressed by the initial lack of contact from her new doctor.

Mrs Quentin felt that the strategies she had developed to combat the uncertainties of living with P.D. had been encouraged, if not subtly initiated, by her GP:

MRS QUENTIN: He pointed out to me a lot of people have it and some of them manage to lead normal lives, because John Betjeman did, didn't he? And he put the ideas into your mind, although I've never discussed it with him fully.... I'm sure he must think the same things, because little things sometimes that I've said to him, and his answers ...

R.P.: They've kind of locked in together?
MRS QUENTIN: That's right.

It did not matter that fears remained unspoken and that GPs' understanding was largely implicit. These patients felt that their GPs really listened and were sensitively attuned to what was going on. They felt understood and cared for as individuals. Even if their distress was couched in more general terms than those discussed earlier in this chapter, these patients felt that their GP knew, as far as anyone not having the illness could know, what it was 'really like'. Such a relationship helped to make the anxieties and distress of the illness experience more bearable.

SUMMARY AND COMMENT

This chapter has explored some of the uncertainties, anxieties and fears which living with P.D. presented, and the routines patients developed to make sense of a life whose predictability had been shaken. The urge to impose order on disorder was as important to patients here as it was in attempting to manage information discovery and the drug regimen. Here their very identities were at stake. Whether strategies reflected an outlook on life that was applied to other life crises or whether they had evolved in response to the particular demands of the illness, they came to constitute a body of expertise with which to make sense of the illness. This expertise enabled patients to be at least partially in control, although, as shown, routines had to be continually rethought as the illness progressed.

Crucially, patients' experiences of handling the inner distress of having P.D. were different from those described by GPs in the previous chapter. Indeed, the uncertainties themselves were different, in as much as they directly affected patients' lives, as opposed to posing problems of how far to become involved in what was work for a GP.

This had important implications for communication. The role patients saw their own GPs playing in supporting their endeavours varied. The absence of support left those patients who wanted help, and found their GP detached, feeling abandoned and fearful. Mis- or non-communication had serious consequences for their ability to handle anxiety. Patients had to turn elsewhere. Often there was nowhere *to* turn.

Patients were more likely to have been helped by those GPs in the study who had a more empathic approach to their work. This was vividly shown by the experiences of those four patients in the study who had the benefits of a supportive relationship. The presence of a caring and understanding GP made an important difference to their lives. Although they talked in terms of 'feeling understood', 'being valued as a person' or of feeling that their GP 'really cared'—nebulous qualities which are difficult to define— these patients were reassured. However, implicitly, their GPs were addressing the fears which haunted them. They had made the imaginative leap from possessing clinical experience of the condition to understanding something of the experience of having P.D. Patients' anxieties could better be contained.

However, some patients did not consider their GP an appropriate figure to consult with such concerns. This is important, considering that the previous chapter showed that some GPs in the study thought that involvement in these areas was an important part of their role. Should GPs be involved in such concerns? Are they the best people to deliver these skills? Patients at least wanted the security of knowing that should they need to talk about their distress, their GPs would be sensitive and responsive. The patient–doctor relationship had to provide a basic framework within which patients could discuss their human concerns on a feeling level. Empathy was crucial.

Doctors need to be especially alert. Patients used a different vocabulary when relating to their GPs from that portrayed earlier in this chapter. They did not describe their terror of becoming wheelchair-bound to their GPs. Fears seemed to be translated into more general terms, such as 'depression' or 'stress', which were considered more appropriate for a doctor, or simply remained unspoken.

Patients' fears were both unique to them and universal. Responses were derived, at least in part, from the wider social and cultural meanings chronic illness holds in our society. But patients' anxieties needed an individual response. There is a world of difference between the experience of suffering uncertainty and being a helping—but necessarily distinct—observer. Some patients showed that GPs could transcend the limitations of their own experience, and understand, in the fullest meaning of the word. In turn, I hope this chapter has provided a deeper appreciation of what it is to be a P.D. patient, so that GPs will be better equipped to respond effectively and sensitively to the P.D. experience.

8
Conclusions: Patient and Doctor—Match and Mismatch

INTRODUCTION

This book tells the story of how patients and doctors experienced and managed the uncertainties of P.D. and how this process may be both cause and consequence of miscommunication between the two. I have explored how a group of P.D. patients and a separate group of GPs viewed P.D. and the implications of these perceptions for building an effective patient–doctor relationship. The book has shown how the struggle to impose order on the disorder raised by the onset of chronic illness may sometimes lead patients and doctors down different paths. They were handling different problems; or, rather, the same initial problem, P.D., had different meanings and consequences for both parties. Some of the uncertainties arose as a result of the clinical features specific to the disease. Others arose from the special difficulties of managing a chronic illness. As I have shown, these were of quite a different order of experience for both parties involved.

For patients, uncertainties were ever present, impinging directly and continuously on their lives. They were struggling to come to terms with the fact that they had contracted a chronic and progressively disabling illness for which there is, at the time of writing, no cure. How were they to make their lives meaningful? They did not know what was going to happen or when, and how the illness would affect their work, family responsibilities and relationships. Crucially, they could not plan ahead. The props on which we all rely to chart our way through life were no longer reliable.

Uncertainties had to be managed if patients were to carry on. The book shows how they developed strategies in response to the specific problems of, for example, the drug regimen, and adapted broader approaches which had stood them in good stead in handling other life crises. Managing uncertainties was a way of accomplishing life in the changed role of a person with P.D.

For doctors, uncertainty had a less global impact. It was generally a more practical problem in that GPs were trying to make their work manageable. They continually had to deal with a variety of patients' troubles and somehow emerge unscathed at the end of the day. They were accomplishing their professional rather than their personal lives. While there was genuine uncertainty about the prognosis for any particular P.D. patient, much more important, I believe, was the uncertainty about what and how much information to share with patients and how to cope with the limitations of strictly medical intervention. Likewise, doctors developed a set of strategies and routines with which to protect themselves from being overwhelmed by their patients' distress. Anxiety only impinged on their own personal lives to the extent that GPs felt threatened or inadequate in the face of their patients' suffering. Mental anguish was the experience of patients rather than of doctors.

How far can GPs help in such a situation? A picture of actual and potential match and mismatch of perspectives has emerged. When patients' feelings had been understood and responded to, encounters with their GPs were seen as satisfying and supportive. The GP was an important figure in helping them come to terms with the illness. Conversely, where this had not happened and there had been no meeting of minds, distress and anxiety for patients were often heightened.

My concern has been with how to bring these disparate experiences closer together so that the patient–doctor relationship may be a source of strength for patients, and clinical experience *with*, and patient experience *of*, the condition may meet at the level of understanding.

The book, therefore, is a plea for understanding, but of a particular kind. Understanding as viewed here is not concerned with the acquisition of facts. Rather it is an art of the imagination, involving putting oneself in another's shoes. Such understanding calls for a reappraisal by doctors of the way they think about their work, of the assumptions they make about patients and of the effect of these judgements on patients' lives. The evidence has shown just how difficult such an exercise is.

It may seem that I am unfairly placing the onus for change on GPs' shoulders. In so far as they have control over the allocation of health service provision, I believe that any constructive remedies must, of necessity, come from them. My talks with them have encouraged me to believe that such a task could be undertaken; doctors were often self-critical about their perceived limitations. They were also critical of their peers. Most were eager to improve their skills. But doctors do not work in a social vacuum. My plea is also for understanding from those who teach, train and work professionally with GPs. The whole framework within which patient care is provided calls for a fresh approach. Patients also have a vital role to play. Greater understanding on their part may help to bring about change.

There are two essential conditions. First, doctors need to equip themselves with a better picture of the way their services look through the eyes of their patients, asking themselves how helpful and relevant their actions are to patients in managing P.D. Second, it is vitally important that doctors understand the nature of the P.D. experience for the patient: what it means to be chronically ill with a long-term, progressively disabling disease in a society which values independence and self-reliance. If these requirements are met, and the book has provided the foundations on which such understandings may grow, I believe that patients and GPs may develop a mutual partnership in managing the disease so that anxiety may be contained and the illness experience made more bearable.

This chapter begins by placing the study in a wider context. I then identify and discuss four broader issues that emerged which have crucial implications for the patient–doctor relationship. These are then examined in relation to the three areas of concern which have been raised in the book—information, drug management, and care rather than cure. The chapter concludes with some suggestions to improve patient care.

THE STUDY AND ITS BROADER CONTEXT

The study was an interpretative exercise. It focused on a small group of patients and doctors: I cannot guarantee, nor did I set out to ensure, that the two groups were demographically typical. What mattered was the context. All patients and all GPs confronted the dilemmas of a chronic illness. In so far as I was probably interviewing more approachable GPs, and most patients had the support of membership of the Parkinson's Disease Society, the conclusions I have reached about the level of mutual understanding between P.D. patients and GPs may be overoptimistic.

I was searching for patterns of response which possessed their own validity as expressions of human experience in a distressing situation. At stake are the reliability and validity with which these expressions have been interpreted. I shall show in the final chapter how I believe this project has adhered to the canons of good scholarship, which are fully as demanding as those of quantitative research.

It is clearly not a definitive analysis. Rather it sets the scene for further enquiry. For example, the scope of the study could be extended to include larger numbers. Its theoretical framework could be developed. Future research might also incorporate a matching exercise which focuses on specific pairings of patients and GPs and explores particular interpersonal relationships.

The usefulness of this study, I believe, lies in its identification of areas where GPs may helpfully redirect their attention. Its interest lies in the nature of the insights which have emerged from concentration on a small group, insights which are unlikely to be tapped by a quantitative approach. Its principal virtue is that it has explored the perspectives of *both* patients and doctors, illuminating areas of difficulty which a focus exclusively on one party would have obscured.

Crucially, the study has important implications for patient–doctor communication in the management of other chronic illnesses. The fact that doctors spontaneously related their discussion of P.D. patients to those with diabetes, M.S., cancer, to the elderly and to the terminally ill indicates that the study has a much wider message. P.D. may well prove to be a useful model in exploring what happens in the management of a whole range of other chronic illnesses with which general practice is increasingly concerned.

CASTING A WIDER NET

A number of broader themes emerged from the study which have implications for interaction between patient and doctor. Stated briefly, they are as follows. First, every patient is a person, a unique individual, behind his/her illness. Second, the illness is not only a physical, but as much or more a psychological and social condition. Third, a closer approximation, if not reconciliation, needs to be sought between the clinical experience of the doctor and the patient's perception of his/her condition. Fourth are the consequences of the above for the patient–doctor relationship and what might be accomplished were it to be viewed differently.

(1) Patients are not simply diseased bodies. Neither are they 'types' of patients, but people who happen to have P.D., one of a variety of statuses, both positive and negative, they hold in life. As such, they have unique needs and wishes which extend far beyond any medical interest in them as disease categories or cases with 'typical' characteristics. A recurrent theme throughout this book has been patients' need for individualized care from their GPs which will give due consideration to these wider aspects of their personalities.

However, there is a fundamental tension here: that between the complexity and variability of patients' responses to uncertainty, on the one hand, and, on the other, GPs' needs to simplify in order to reduce ambiguity and process their work smoothly.

Although the medical literature impresses on doctors that 'no two cases are alike' (Stern and Lees, 1982), the study showed that in practice they sometimes caused distress to their patients by the routine way in which they treated them. The use of broad, unverified judgements by some doctors and the confidence with which these were often asserted tended to get in the way of their treating patients as individuals. Of course, flexibility complicated life for doctors. The nearer they came to responding to patients as individuals, the more they felt that they risked exposing themselves to those very uncertainties which they found so difficult to handle. Such a dilemma is not unresolvable, as the evidence of some patients' accounts of their GPs has shown, but it does require doctors to take risks and to cope with the attendant anxiety.

I am not, of course, questioning the need for doctors to make judgements; rather the contrary. I am arguing that doctors need to develop finer, more perceptive and sensitive judgements which would provide a greater knowledge of the patient as person. This is only possible if doctors understand what is likely to be happening when patients are faced with the need to come to terms with the implications of having P.D.

(2) While I have been concerned to explore responses at the individual level, the emergence of certain patterns of response suggested that I was also confronting problems which derive from the wider social and cultural background of which patients and doctors are a part. Patients' experience with and doctors' handling of P.D. take place in a broader social arena where the meanings of chronic illness are played out.

On one level, patients talked about the impact of the illness on their everyday lives, their work, their marriages and their friends. Doctors need to see that these are areas of life which are vitally important in understanding patients' responses to the uncertainties of the illness. However, as Schneider and Conrad (1983) have pointed out, social and psychological phenomena are not just factors, variables to the situation which may be plucked from the air and treated as discrete entities. Illness is itself a social and cultural phenomenon. However, I do not share those authors' pessimism about the likelihood of physicians being able to respond to the psychological and social sequelae of chronic illness. The evidence from some patients in the study has shown that such a response is possible. Their GPs *did* attend to such concerns.

On another level, patients' feelings and beliefs, although unique to them, were at the same time socially and culturally patterned. Chronic illness evokes very specific images which threaten the norms of self-sufficiency and physical and economic independence so highly prized in our society. Terror of being wheelchair-bound, for example, is not just an isolated individual response. It is part of the wider body of social attitudes towards chronic illness and dependence (well documented by, for example, Helman, 1984; Anderson and Bury, 1988; Williams and Wood, 1988). Further, the patients' and GPs' strategies I have described are both individual responses and are part of our culturally shared ways of dealing with anxiety and distress. Paradoxically, the individual must be placed within a wider social context if a genuinely personal approach is to be achieved. To treat the patient out of context is to depersonalize him/her.

Again the tension for doctors was apparent. In developing a broader understanding of their work with patients, GPs risked exposing themselves to uncertainties which could complicate matters. Confining their concerns to the management of P.D. at a clinical level only was comparatively safe. They were on their home ground. Yet, for those who possessed it, a wider knowledge and understanding enabled doctors to target their services more appropriately. They needed to understand in order to reduce the very uncertainty which they feared.

(3) Third, the study raises the question of the difference between doctors' possession of clinical knowledge as a body of facts and patients' direct experience of the illness, a question which must be the starting-point for any study which seeks to explore communication between the two. The debate on this issue has recently centred on the disparity between lay and medical explanatory models of the illness (see, for example, Blumhagen, 1980; Helman, 1984; Tuckett *et al.*, 1985). I should like to broaden it further. GPs seeking to help P.D. patients are faced with the problem of how to overcome the limitations of their own individual experience. We can, of course, only experience our own lives. We can never completely know another's experiences. Nevertheless, we can view others' worlds if only in 'snapshots'. This involves the development of empathy, a fellow-feeling for those in pain, and the ability to respond to the patient as another human being. We may not be the patient, but we may better share the experience of what it is like by the cultivation of an 'as if I were you' approach. Wilmer (1987, p. 207) describes the process: 'We borrow his feelings, look at them, feel and understand them. We do not take them; we only enter them to understand how he feels.' It involves the capacity both to share and to stand back in order to be able to help. The basic ingredient is imagination, which invites the question whether this is a quality people are born with or whether it may be acquired, an issue I address in the section on recommendations.

So much may be obvious. At the end of the day, this may not take us very far. The exercise of goodwill may be taken for granted. Doctors in this study showed that they had it in abundance. Yet many patients found that things still went awry. It is not just a doctor's niceness that is at issue. Doctors in the study said that they had found how difficult it was to be compassionate—and to sustain this—with their P.D. patients.

The problem again is that the development of empathy risks exposing doctors to anxieties and fears they may prefer to avoid. It can be intensely threatening to enter the feeling world of another. However, if the patient–doctor relationship is to be positive, the doctor needs to share and understand, if only fleetingly, what it must be like to have P.D.

(4) Fourth, if these issues are to be tackled, a reformulation of the patient–GP relationship along more egalitarian lines is needed. With Tuckett *et al.* (1985), I believe that patients and doctors may become partners, jointly engaged in managing the disease and drug regimen as 'third parties', as it were, with mutual respect for each other's com-

plementary skills. Patients need to be encouraged to help doctors to formulate what the problems, as they see them, are, and, as far as possible, share in subsequent decision-making. This is particularly important in the management of chronic illnesses, which are, by definition, often complex and protracted.

Meeting patients half-way also requires doctors to re-evaluate the balance of control within the relationship. Tuckett *et al.* (1985) have found the GPs they studied uncomfortable with, and unwilling to give up, being in charge. Yet the management of a long-term chronic illness such as P.D. calls for a dialogue between the parties as co-participants, not as between passive patient and paternalistic doctor. Doctors will need to reassess how much they need to be in control if they are to empower their patients, and to confront the hesitation and initial anxiety they may feel in delegating varying degrees of responsibility to patients. It is a matter of respecting the patient as having complementary rather than inferior skills. A doctor's skill is of little use if it does not engage patients' expertise. This study has shown how detailed and sophisticated patients' knowledge of their illness and its treatment is. Patients' expertise may, in fact, give doctors confidence rather than detract from it.

In the light of these broader issues, I shall review the findings under the three headings identified in the book: information, drug management, and care rather than cure.

MATCH AND MISMATCH

Information

The broader issues discussed above are brought into sharp relief by the necessity for doctors to explain, and for patients to understand from doctors, what a diagnosis entails. Doctors were faced with a translation exercise, the outcome of which they could not gauge with any certainty. Explanations could either be treated as a discrete body of facts, to be disclosed or not according to the judgements GPs held about their patients, or as a jointly negotiated task of helping to convert the facts into an understanding which was meaningful to patients. The two approaches are very different activities.

Not surprisingly, some GPs in the study were reluctant to become involved in the tricky area of helping patients to interpret the facts: fearful of what unforeseen consequences might follow if they did so; hopeful, perhaps, that other events might supervene, making detailed explanations 'unnecessary'. Communication could be simplified and standardized.

These doctors tended to develop a house style to suit all comers, based on assumptions about age, intelligence and emotional stability. The weight of importance given to age as a category was particularly striking and illustrated the great difficulty younger doctors had in empathizing with the elderly sick. The use of such broad judgements helped to reduce the need for individual decisions. With the best of intentions, patients were protected from the impact of potentially distressing information. Patients remained patients, rather than emerging as persons.

However, if information is given only to 'the emotionally stable', 'the more intelligent' and 'younger patients', how do anxious, less intelligent and older patients fare? It cannot be assumed that they, too, do not want to control the process of accepting the implications of having P.D.

It was what the facts meant for patients' lives that mattered, as Dr Quinn in his new-found role as carer all too painfully discovered. Patients' uncertainties were of quite a different order. Where they felt that their needs to understand the facts were not being addressed, frustration and anxiety were aggravated. Conversely, where patients felt that their GPs were attentive to the meanings P.D. held for them, and were able to cross the divide which separates first-hand from indirect experience, the process of finding out what to expect was transformed. Patients' and doctors' concerns matched. Patients felt understood as persons, with their own unique needs and priorities, rather than placed in predetermined categories.

After diagnosis, patients faced the difficult task of imposing order on what was a new and potentially disturbing event, whose impact on their lives could as yet be only dimly discerned. Patients' reactions were much more complex, it seemed, than some doctors appreciated. Understanding for patients was a dynamic process, spread out over time and, indeed, never ending. For communication between patient and doctor to be effective, there needed to be a continuous dialogue, constantly evolving in line with patients' changing needs. Moreover, patients tried to manage the uncertainties involved in understanding what to expect in ways which often transcended doctors' judgements. Levels of intelligence, educational attainment, age and emotional stability were most unreliable guides to predicting what patients did or did not want to know. Indeed, the study included two patients, both highly educated and intelligent, who deliberately chose not to know the implications of the illness. Knowledge of what the clinical facts meant was not always the priceless resource other writers on patient–doctor communication have suggested. Sometimes it was too threatening. A GP needs to understand the diversity of response and its changing nature over time: in fact, mentally to address the very complexity which might arouse anxiety. He/she can not operate effectively and sensitively with a fixed set of expectations about patients' needs. Some patients were content to live in the present, others not so: again imagination may be the key.

Other doctors in the study understood that uncertainty of this nature could be *reduced* by a more open policy. Doctors needed to know what their patients were feeling about P.D. and what the onset of the illness was going to mean for their lives in order to target their explanations most appropriately. Far from increasing uncertainty, feedback enabled them to see whether they were on course or not. A more open approach allowed GPs to respond both to those who wanted information and to those who did not. Where explaining was seen as a two-way process and the patient–GP relationship as a forum where the two parties could exchange complementary knowledge, these GPs were able to meet their patients more than half-way.

The Drugs

The management of the drug regimen particularly focuses attention on the nature of the patient–GP relationship and whether this might more usefully be formulated along mutual partnership rather than traditional, paternalistic lines.

GPs had differing ideas about how far patients should be encouraged to monitor and adjust their daily treatment themselves. Their views were based, as before, on their varying assessments of patients' competence. Some GPs felt less anxious when they were nominally in charge. They were uncertain as to how patients might react to the discovery that the drugs had unpleasant side-effects which, over time, might become difficult to manage. They preferred to keep these uncertainties to themselves. Also, retention of control over treatment meant that GPs were on comparatively safe ground. Managing medication was a well-established part of a GP's repertoire of skills. However, other GPs in the study found that anxiety was reduced all round by sharing management. They were less worried about the possible effects on patients when they discovered that the medication had its limitations. Patients were not led astray by expectations which might subsequently be difficult for doctors to justify. Anxieties were shared. When responsibility for the daily management of treatment was the situation in which most patients ultimately found themselves, was control, sharing or some intermediate compromise likely to be most helpful to patients?

Some patients were intensely frustrated and rendered anxious by the discovery that *they* as much as their doctors had to be experts in assessing the effects of the medication on them, particularly in the absence of firm yardsticks as to how they should feel. Not all patients wanted such a responsibility. Others responded to the situation with alacrity and found that self-management enhanced their confidence. Development of expertise was a means of controlling anxiety, as many studies on chronic illness have shown (see, for example, Strauss and Glaser, 1975; Strauss *et al.*, 1985; Anderson and Bury, 1988). However, patients' responses again bore little relationship to the broader assumptions held by some doctors about patients' competence. Age, intelligence and emotional stability were inadequate pointers as to how patients reacted to this unexpected challenge. The reality was a great deal more complex.

An understanding of the social context in which patients had to manage the drug regimen was vitally important for doctors. Drugs were not simply things people took. Being on medication for life had profound meanings for patients relating to wider social and cultural beliefs about taking drugs. Drug dependence, or 'being an addict', as Mrs Jenson described her husband, was often distressing for patients—a fact few felt their own GPs or consultants appreciated.

The programme of treatment also has to be woven into the fabric of people's lives. While it is not so with many other drugs, the administration of these had to be planned. Such planning required constant monitoring of one's bodily reactions. As Mrs Pembridge reminds us, 'It's not a case of taking one tablet twice a day'. Treatment also constantly reminded patients of their condition. In a very real sense medication *was* P.D. Doctors need to understand this world, to appreciate how their instructions, or the absence of explicit instructions, have to be translated into a viable way of managing life for patients.

Most patients in the study found that advice from their GPs was of marginal relevance in helping with the drug management—a finding at variance with the active and informed role many GPs in the study considered they played. Yet doctors in the study evidently found it difficult to help to translate pharmacological knowledge into a workable regimen for patients. This, together with the failure of some patients' GPs to appreciate the wider social context in which patients lived out their lives, may account for the lack of preparation given to patients for assuming responsibility for their treatment. Most doctors in the study were reluctant to be specific with their information. Little guidance seemed available to alert patients to the fact that chronic illness and its treatment could not be managed in the same way as acute illnesses, with which patients were generally more familiar. Little seemed to have been done to ease the transition from compliant recipient to more active initiator. Patients were often left to find out for themselves how to manage the regimen in a way which was consistent with their other priorities, as Mr Dempsey so engagingly illustrated. Patients could not exercise choice without the tools to do so. Gaining knowledge the hard way was often filled with anxiety. There was a mismatch between doctors' interests and patients' needs.

A flexible response to management seems to be the way forward. The question is not one of GPs *either* maintaining control or sharing with the patient, but of the adoption of various mixes between the two, tailored according to patients' individual needs. At various times in the course of the illness, patients needed greater or lesser degrees of support. Again doctors need to understand how their patients are feeling if they are to help to balance the medication effectively. An open approach by them might arouse uncertainty; alternatively, attentiveness to what patients are saying, and a knowledge of them as persons situated within a web of other social relationships, may help GPs to know whether they are on course or not.

Care Rather Than Cure

Caring for P.D. patients poses a difficult dilemma for doctors: How can they best help their patients without themselves becoming emotionally drained and overwhelmed? How close can they get to understanding what the experience of P.D. is really like and yet emerge intact at the end of the day? Just being there, acknowledging the limitations of strictly medical intervention, exposed GPs to the raw experience of what P.D. meant. It could plunge them into a frightening world where they did not know their way. Not all GPs in the study thought that they either could or should be involved in patients' deeper concerns. Some adopted a more detached approach, focusing on the clinical matters at hand, as a safer option. Others favoured a more open approach and thought that, within limits, such involvement was an important part of general practice. Indeed, medicine would be very dull without it, as Dr Leadbrough noted. Involvement served doctors' needs. They were able to empathize, however transitorily, with what it must be like. However, their anxieties were at one remove from those of their patients. Therein lay the greatest source of mismatch.

For patients, by contrast, their very identities were at stake. Life was a constant struggle to maintain their integrity against a continuous process of erosion of their physical (and sometimes mental) selves. In the task of making sense of P.D., the two parties were engaged in very different activities which would bring them closer together or cause them to move further apart, according to the manner in which they were conducted.

Not all patients considered their own GPs to be the most appropriate person with whom ·to share these concerns. Some had the support of friends and relatives; others, however, struggled in isolation. Where patients wanted such support from their GPs and failed to obtain it, anxiety and distress were magnified. Where depression, for example, was responded to at a clinical rather than at a personal level, patients felt rebuffed. They wanted to engage their doctors as human beings rather than simply as mechanical dispensers of prescriptions. Conversely, empathy from their GPs made a crucial difference to the quality of other patients' lives. They were understood as persons. Their GPs had some feeling for what it meant to have P.D. and for the importance of the social setting in which patients lived. Patients' and doctors' concerns were at one.

Ultimately, of course, patients must deal with fear and despair themselves. But do they have to feel so totally alone? Is not an understanding ally precisely what a GP can—and in some cases did—provide? Patients will vary, of course, in the amount, nature and timing of the support they require. But I believe that the very nature of a chronic illness such as P.D. makes some level of involvement desirable, so long as the patient wishes it. Again what is needed is a sensitive approach, one that is both attuned to those patients for whom discussion of such matters would be an intrusion on their privacy, and alert and receptive to those who, though they may not always express it as such, were often desperate for support.

Finally, for communication to be effective, there needs to be a meeting of minds. Clinical experience with the condition may be linked with direct experience of the illness at the level of understanding as I have viewed it. GPs need to know something of what it means to be physically dependent on others, rather than responding to patients simply as diseased bodies or types of cases. Again some doctors found that sharing patients' concerns, however momentarily, helped to allay uncertainty all round. Doctors better understood the nature of the difficulties they were confronting. Indeed, a few doctors in the study had developed special skills to enable them to respond more sensitively.

The fragility of patients' attempts to control the anxieties of managing life with P.D. also indicates the need for continuing receptivity on the part of GPs. Effective support is a dynamic process. It merits much more than a one-off response. The idea of patient and doctor learning to manage the disease together as allies means that GPs have something important to learn from patients. The notion of GP-as-learner is perhaps difficult for GPs to accept, but it is a vitally important step if the patient–GP relationship is to become a supportive partnership where communication may flourish.

* * * * * *

If GPs are to play a positive role in the lives of their P.D. patients (and I believe that they both can and should), they need to understand those anxieties and fears that are likely to be troubling patients and to appreciate that the way they manage their own, less direct, uncertainties may not always be helpful to patients. Where doctors are able to address patients' need to find meaning in an event as arbitrary as the onset of P.D., such understanding holds out rich possibilities for patient care. It has the potential to transform the P.D. experience for patients from one of anxiety and distress to one of a life crisis made manageable with support.

Having identified the needs and placed the findings in a wider context, I shall finally look at what might usefully be done. How, in practical terms, can doctors transcend the limitations of their own experience and treat a patient as a person?

RECOMMENDATIONS

Like the GP, I find it difficult to reach for a prescription pad. There are no miracle answers. Nevertheless, this research provides some indications of the lines along which GPs may usefully work. I am not underestimating the difficulties GPs face. There are many factors in general practice militating against the suggestions I am able to make, not least the practical pressure of heavy caseloads. Moreover, my suggestions are, in the final analysis, simply instruments. The use of instruments without the development of understanding is of little value. However, with the understanding as I have outlined it, GPs may better be able to use those appropriate to the situations which cause most difficulty.

Care for the chronic sick demands a very special kind of expertise. Yet the distinctive problems of supporting the chronically ill have not received the attention which has, for example, recently been developed in caring for the terminally ill. Paradoxically, chronic illness is perhaps more difficult to manage sensitively and effectively than terminal illness. There is no immediate end in sight. Support needs to be sustained over a lengthy period, and over a series of gradually worsening situations. If GPs are the best people to give this support (and most GPs in the study felt that they wanted to do so, at any rate as part of a team), then I believe that more could be done to prepare them for this task than is currently the case. There are five areas which merit attention.

First, inexperience of P.D., about which patients often complained, is relatively easily remedied. Teaching needs to concentrate less on the skills of differential diagnosis in obscure neurological complaints and focus on the more common conditions, such as P.D., which a GP is likely to meet in his/her work. Neurology was sometimes seen as a rarefied discipline.

Several GPs suggested that consultants might hold regular sessions at their surgeries to keep them briefed. Such a move, in turn, might help to rectify the lack of confidence which may have hampered the GPs of some patients in the study. Teaching also needs to focus more on the management of the chronically ill as a process. Despite some attempts to shift the emphasis, the balance between care and cure in medical education is still not adequately geared to the task of sustaining care over time for the chronic sick (see, for example, Sanson-Fisher and Maguire, 1980; Tuckett *et al.*, 1985; Ridsdale, personal communication, 1986).

Second, better liaison with consultants all round is needed. GPs themselves sometimes commented on the lack of effective co-ordination. More thought needs to be given to spelling out exactly what 'joint partnership' means in practice. This cannot be achieved where GPs feel that consultants have insufficient confidence in their complementary expertise.

Third, chronic illness requires much more home-based care than is at present the case. I am aware that I am moving against the tide in suggesting this, but the trend towards situating general practice in intermediate centres between the home and the hospital favours the doctor at the expense of the patient. Patients frequently said how much they wanted their GPs to 'pop in just to see how you're getting on' on a fairly regular basis, rather than merely responding to medical emergencies. Chronic illness is lived largely in the home. I believe that such exposure to patients' lives would also help doctors to appreciate more fully what it means to have P.D.—an understanding which is more difficult to achieve in the impersonal surroundings of the surgery.

The fourth area is the most difficult. I cannot claim to be able to lay down recipes to improve those intangibles in personal relationships which facilitate better communication. There is no short course in developing the necessary skills of perceptiveness and sensitivity. In a sense, they are the work of a lifetime. Nevertheless, I believe that the development of basic counselling techniques and skills in self-awareness may provide doctors with the opportunity to not only examine their own feelings of helplessness and inadequacy, but also explore how keeping these very understandable feelings under control may create difficulties for the very patients they are trying to help. I am asking, no less, that doctors be encouraged to scrutinize the values and beliefs on which they base their work. I am not suggesting that GPs should become counsellors but that training in the skills of understanding and learning how, as much as what, to think are the essence of sensitive communication with patients.

I do not subscribe to the view that such skills are innate and, if lacking, cannot be acquired. Thompson (1984), reviewing the results of training programmes to date, found that while there was considerable room for improvement, 'the ingredients of the interview' could be taught. Maguire and Faulkner's more recent work (1988) in teaching medical personnel to deal more sensitively with their cancer patients found that such training is not only feasible, but also effective. One key to success may lie in targeting training programmes to the difficulties posed by managing special patient groups. This study has shown how difficult some younger doctors found the task of relating to older patients. Improved training in working with the elderly, who will constitute an increasing part of a GP's caseload, would be a timely move. Such training is not a soft option to be tacked on to the end of medical training as a concession to liberal ideas. It is fundamental.

Fifth, the process of understanding does not, of course, end there. What is needed is a systematic, on-going programme geared to doctors' own evolving needs. Like those of everyone else, doctors' perceptions change with experience. Further, the emotionally demanding nature of caring for the chronically sick suggests that there is a need, as in other caring professions, to support the supporters. The medical curriculum still leaves students very much on their own to come to terms with the emotional pressures of caring for those in distress (Weston and Lipkin, 1989). Yet GPs in the study who had such support felt better equipped to cope with the demands involved in caring for their P.D. patients.

Last but not least, patients may also contribute to change. Faced with GPs who were inexperienced in dealing with P.D. and apparently unwilling to rectify this, patients were often fearful of being 'struck-off' if they tried to change their GPs. They may feel more confident knowing that GPs do not take it as a personal affront if one of their patients wishes to change. Dr Fleming, for example, was astonished when I told him of the anxiety changing GPs had caused Mr and Mrs Canning.

Nevertheless, patients are developing a stronger consumer voice. My reservations about patient participation groups stem from the fact that they are usually organized *by* doctors *for* patients, rather than by patients themselves, and fail to attract those most in need of support. While the initiative may come from doctors, the strategy should be to hand autonomy over to patients, allowing them to be in charge. I also believe that the Parkinson's Disease Society may play a vital role in encouraging patients to pool their resources and to promote greater awareness of the standards they should expect from their own GPs. In this, my findings have very positive implications for the further development of current initiatives. Such expectations often have a way of fulfilling themselves. Patients, too, have much to understand.

This brings me full circle to my point of departure: the vital importance for GPs of an in-depth understanding of what it is like to have a chronic illness. This, I believe, is the key to better communication. Armed with such an appreciation, GPs may better be able to help their patients and minimize the uncertainty and its effects which so often detracted from the quality of patients' lives. I am well aware that such understanding does not emerge simply from reading a book. It calls for a considerable effort of the imagination and sustained work on the part of its readers. The GPs in the study impressed me with their care and concern and their desire to be of help. I feel confident that they and their colleagues will want to give serious thought to ways of improving their relationships with P.D. and other chronically ill patients. If it is true that patients need to be seen as persons, then it is equally true of doctors. That is the inspiration behind this book.

9
Doing Research: More Than an Afterthought

INTRODUCTION

Health care professionals, GPs and patients themselves may be unfamiliar with the approach I have used. I need to be explicit and honest about the way the research was conducted, how it affected the patients and GPs involved, and how my thoughts and feelings about it changed over time. This involves a degree of systematic reflection on my part which may strike some as unnecessary or even self-indulgent. The intricate relationship between researcher, researched and research process may be strange to those accustomed to regard research as a neutral activity. It is not. The researcher is a dynamic part of the research, and his/her attitudes, values and feelings cannot be suspended, as it were, in the process. As Berg (1988, p. 226) eloquently argues: '. . . the emotional dynamics in research relationships are an important variable in the social science research process. They are not merely sources of bias or reactivity, but rather the context in which research happens, influencing both the process and the outcome.' Moreover, feelings and attitudes change cumulatively with each encounter. To assume otherwise is to obscure what happens when people come together (Wynne, 1988).

These beliefs and feelings need to be thoroughly scrutinized as part of the research process. A study such as this is dependent for its rigour on such an exercise. It must form part of the research account. Self-examination provides future researchers with a firm basis for replication, and it also enables readers to check on the data and draw their own conclusions.

I do not wish to add to the overworked debate about the relative merits of qualitative and quantitative research. The crucial question is the kind of knowledge which I wanted to obtain. My emphasis throughout has been on eliciting meanings, interpretations and experiences. Given these objectives, questions of randomness or typicality, although vitally important for some research, were less so here. The analysis does not focus on the particular characteristics of patients and doctors, nor does it seek to establish the precise proportions of patients in the population who were satisfied or dissatisfied with their GPs. Rather, I was trying to understand something of the experiences likely to be shared by most patients and doctors faced with the disease, and to draw out themes which emerged from this. My interest was in problems, not proportions.

However, I do not believe my findings are misleadingly atypical. There was no reason to suppose that the impressions and perceptions illustrated here would differ significantly from those of patients and GPs in the population at large. I should have been alerted to the existence of such bias had the results, for example, been overwhelmingly negative or critical among the patients. This was not the case. The cases studied here were, I believe, representative in the more colloquial sense in that they illuminated important areas of patients' and GPs' ideas and experiences which have more general applicability.

My aim was to elicit a different kind of knowledge from that obtainable from survey techniques. Thus the use of prestructured questionnaires, attitude and rating scales, or reliance on preformulated hypotheses, were simply inappropriate for this task. A different method was required. I have therefore used those research tools which are most sensitive to qualitative analysis, namely semi-structured interviewing (my main research instrument) and some direct observation. Such interviewing allows subjects the freedom to explain what they want to say and, critically, to talk about those aspects of a topic the researcher may not have considered. The two kinds of knowledge and, therefore, their respective methods, are not in competition. Ideally they are complementary. I believe the approach I have used yields rich insights into what I consider to be a neglected field: how patients and GPs think about 'the same' disease and how this may affect encounters between them.

This chapter describes first the more conventional problems of negotiating access and establishing criteria for selection, and the procedures used in interviewing patients and doctors. Second, I have tried to broaden the discussion. There is space to address only one of the many fascinating issues which occur in any research but a particularly significant one here: the intricate relationship between involvement and responsibility and the question of power.

However, two problems arose almost immediately I embarked on the project: one practical, which was resolved fairly quickly; the other theoretical, which stayed with me—and rightly so—throughout the process of conducting and writing about the research.

SETTING THE SCENE

The Matching Question

First was the problem of matching patient with doctor. The first three patients I approached were reluctant to allow me to interview their own GPs, perhaps fearing that their accounts would be given less credence. Studying individual pairs of particular patients and doctors was not going to be feasible—a problem I had only partly anticipated.

This led to a major shift in the formulation of the research which working within the present model allows one to make. I turned to what proved to be a much richer exercise: the mapping of attitudes of patients and doctors across a whole range of encounters within the particular context of P.D. Specific interpersonal interplay was no longer important. My context was P.D. I was comparing what patients with P.D. needed and expected from their GPs (and what they thought they obtained) with GPs' perceptions of what their own P.D. patients wanted or needed. It was a serendipitous discovery. Had I restricted myself to studying specific pairings, I would have been dealing with single-instance inferences. This would have required a much larger sample than I had originally proposed from which to draw valid conclusions about the nature of interpersonal communication, restricting the depth of understanding I could have achieved. Instead I have been concerned with generalizable evidence which can be distilled from a number of individual accounts. Such an emphasis positively called for in-depth interviews with small groups. The focus was on understanding, not corroboration. We need to understand the meanings underlying human behaviour before we can attempt to account for it.

Why Uncertainty?

The second problem is essential to any piece of research: that of continuously testing, rejecting, modifying and refining one's interpretations of the data. Out of all the possible constructions that might have been placed on what was happening when patients and doctors talked about their ideas and experiences, why this particular explanation, especially when it was not always readily apparent?

It was the position from which I started. I knew from other studies, as well as from personal experience, that people with M.S. found uncertainty particularly difficult to live with. However, as I collected people's stories and familiarized myself more with the literature, other explanations suggested themselves and the question of uncertainty was, for a time, dropped. It was doctors' accounts which particularly bothered me. Doctors were trying to establish boundaries to their work, yes. They were understandably reluctant to be drawn into difficult positions, such as having to break bad news to their patients. They were anxious to protect themselves, certainly, but from what?

It was tempting and fashionable to interpret the data in terms of the inequalities of power between patient and doctor. However, this did not seem adequately to account for their concerns. It was much too crude. The disparity between lay and medical models of illness had a great deal more to offer. It was clear that patients and doctors thought about the same disease in quite different ways. But it was more specific than that. There was something more fundamental at issue.

It was much easier to identify the reason for patients' concerns. Their stories readily showed that they were beset with uncertainties, fears and apprehension as one problem after another arose which had to be dealt with if they were to carry on. It was the 'dealing with' that finally triggered the connection. Could what was happening to patients also mirror, in different ways, what was preoccupying doctors? The more I looked at this possibility, the more it appeared that doctors were also faced with anxieties—which varied enormously in nature and degree compared with those of patients, but were nonetheless there, as the book has shown. Everything fell into place.

Of course, this does not preclude other interpretations from being made. This is a task I leave to readers. The point is that the very explicitness of this methodological approach allows readers to judge for themselves the value of my analytic framework. This particular interpretation has, to my mind, the closest fit with what patients and doctors sought to convey and is, I believe, pivotal to an understanding of the patient–doctor relationship in the management of chronic illness.

FINDING MY PATIENTS AND OBTAINING ACCOUNTS

I wanted to include as diverse a range of people as possible, so the criteria for selection were broadly framed. Apart from excluding those in residential care as possibly being too ill to take part, the only restrictions made were geographical ones. Interviews were largely, but not exclusively, held within the Greater London area.

Selection

I had not intended to use the Parkinson's Disease Society as a source of patients. I wanted to explore how patients who did not have the benefits of the resources offered by the Society thought about their GPs. I therefore compiled a wide-ranging list of possible places where patients might be found, which included local Crossroads schemes, the local Health Authority, local Friendship Clubs and local branches of Age Concern, and systematically worked through it. However, finding such patients was more difficult than I had foreseen, and, it transpired, all but one of the fifteen turned out to be members of the Society. Either the organizations I approached singled them out as 'interesting cases' (Mr Irving) or Society members were more eager research subjects than others.

Eventually, successful referral sources were three general practitioners (three patients), and two Social Service Department Day Centres (two patients). Four patients were 'snow-ballers' (friends of patients already contacted) and I approached one directly. The remaining five were recruited from local branches of the Society and from the Society's Headquarters.

The Group

Although typicality was not at issue, readers may be interested in some of the main characteristics of the patient group (further details of which are in Appendix 1). I obtained a fairly good cross-section of patients as regards age, age of onset of the illness and degree of impairment, but have probably underrepresented those from Social Classes IV and V. All but one patient, either currently or previously, had been in contact with a consultant neurologist. At the time of first interview, eight patients were consultant-only managed, four were managed by both consultant and GP, and three were GP-only managed. All but two patients who worked flexitime were retired (five patients had retired on health grounds). Ten patients lived with their spouses and family, and five lived on their own. Four patients and the wife of one patient died during the course of the study. One patient got married.

Procedure

Patients were approached first by letter, briefly outlining the aims of the study and assuring them that no information would be passed on to their own doctors—a precaution that turned out to be important. Some patients worried about this at first.

I thought that it would help to focus patients' accounts if I had some idea of their overall evaluations of their GPs. Patients were asked to tick a card saying whether they found their current GP 'very helpful', 'moderately helpful' or 'unhelpful'. Eight patients ticked 'very helpful', four of whom, it transpired, had serious reservations. Mr Canning, for example, later said of his response: 'This must be qualified as within the limits of what he's capable of offering which isn't very much. It's a case of a single comment not being adequate.' Three patients found their GPs 'moderately helpful', one of whom qualified his judgement later, saying 'I find him less helpful now than when I ticked your card' (Mr Irving). Three patients found their GPs 'unhelpful', one of whom changed her judgement when she moved to sheltered accommodation, saying 'At last he's got the message' (Mrs Pembridge). Another changed his GP (Mr Mitchell). One patient was unable to give an assessment (Mr Grenville).

Patient satisfaction is not a stable situation. It changes over time, a process to which qualitative research is uniquely responsive. Had I been content with a simple response, the picture would have been misleading. Moreover, as Locker and Dunt (1978) and Fitzpatrick and Hopkins (1983) have suggested, global evaluations on their own tend to overestimate patient levels of satisfaction. When I asked about specific aspects of their care, I obtained a very different picture.

Interviews

The interviews were carried out mostly in patients' homes. Spouses helped to translate where patients had speech difficulties (four patients). The translation itself is, of course, an added problem. I treated spouses' contributions more as an additional source of data than an accurate representation of what husband or wife intended to convey.

Initially I tried using a totally unstructured approach with two couples who were referred to me by my own GP, one of whom was later included in the study, but this was inhibiting. People expected some structure. Moreover, there were issues I wanted to raise. On the other hand, a detailed Interview Guide which I drew up, was much too restrictive. I found that I did not need to ask many questions: answers flowed from the conversation. I therefore used the Guide only as a basis for discussion, focusing on broad topics. Patients were encouraged to range as widely and divergently over the themes as they wished. They could choose how much—or how little—they wanted to say on any given topic.

Sixty-eight formal interviews were completed, with patients being seen, on average, four times. They took place initially over a fifteen-month period but in most cases there was some form of follow-up—by phone, letter or direct contact—at varying periods over the next three years. Each interview lasted a minimum of one and a half hours and some for much longer. I often spent many hours in patients' homes. The interviews produced some seventy hours of tape-recorded conversation which was transcribed, unedited, yielding some seven hundred pages of typed material. Finally, I asked patients to complete a brief Fact Sheet which provided basic sociodemographic data.

Transcripts were returned to patients for their comments. This was not always what had been expected. Mrs Jenson, for example, said: 'We thought you'd put us with others and sort of *explained*, not this!' Explaining came later. For most patients, this consultation proved to be one of the most valuable parts of the study. Some did want to alter things—the emphasis here, a detail there. They felt responsible for their accounts and wanted to get them 'absolutely right'. Comments such as those of Mrs Quentin ('I hadn't wanted to give the impression that . . .') demonstrated the need to consult those patients who wanted this with material I had explained—a policy to which I have tried to adhere both in this book and elsewhere. It was important to check that, in providing a broader framework for analysis, I had remained faithful to patients' intentions.

GPs: AN ENTRY INTO A DIFFERENT WORLD

Gaining access to GPs was also difficult, but I had expected this. My efforts were conducted against a chorus of comments such as 'as a non-medical person you'll never get any' (local dispensing chemist) or 'the most you'll get will be ten minutes' (GP). This may reflect the 'market research' image with which, Dr Fleming told me, GPs are familiar. In the event, access was less difficult than anticipated and I obtained, and successfully interviewed, eighteen GPs.

Selection

The main criterion used in selecting GPs for interview was their declared experience in caring for P.D. patients, as otherwise we should have been talking hypothetically. (However, this meant that I was probably selecting out those GPs who were seen by patients as being unfamiliar with the illness.) Experience turned out to be fairly limited, with an average of three or four patients per list. Dr Ogilvie, a trainee, had made only one visit to a patient, and, as it transpired, Dr Quinn and Dr Leadbrough had no experience at all with P.D. patients. However, their ability to draw comparisons and contrasts with similar conditions was so telling that their inclusion added greatly to the value of the study.

Sources of referral were varied. Conferences were a happy hunting-ground and I obtained my first five GPs there. First impressions were obviously important. Dr Naughton, for instance, said that he had agreed to see me 'because you seemed to have a human approach'. Meeting GPs beforehand in this way made an enormous difference to the ease of subsequent interviews. It also allowed me to observe GPs operating in settings other than the surgery, thus providing additional checks on the validity of my interpretations.

A personal contact at a London teaching hospital provided three GPs. I obtained a further five contacts from a GP at a local practice. I had negotiated an entrée there with the help of the receptionist—a procedure used with some success by Dowie (1983)—but I discarded it thankfully when sufficient GPs had been selected. It was reminiscent of selling double glazing, and my first attempt had been refused. 'Snowballers' arising from such contacts gave me the remainder of the group.

The Group

Personal details of the group may be found in Appendix 2. It contained four women GPs who combined general practice work with teaching. It also included a high proportion of young GPs (again I had expected this). These 'biases' had distinct advantages. Younger GPs and those responsible for their teaching and training are likely to be in the vanguard of change. The group probably represents the most aware end of the spectrum. Yet the findings have shown that there were still grounds for disquiet.

Procedure

Individual letters were sent to each GP requesting, or confirming, their initial agreement to an interview. The letters briefly explained the aims of the study, stressed the confidentiality of the interview and requested the use of a tape recorder. I explained that I could not write down their comments fast enough and, moreover, was hard of hearing. I wanted to concentrate on listening. GPs were also asked to make a note of P.D. patients on their list, so that we could anchor our talk to specific examples. A letter of introduction from Mrs Mary Baker, Welfare Director of the Parkinson's Disease Society, established my bona fides.

Interviews

Interviews were centred around broad themes which patients, interviewed first, had indicated were of central importance to them. They lasted a minimum of forty-five minutes (except in the case of Dr Ogilvie, who was pressed by his Principal to stand in, where time was slightly curtailed; I have included him as he was the one trainee in the group, fresh from medical school). Some interviews lasted appreciably longer where GPs were interested in pursuing a particular topic. I therefore extended the minimum time limit to one hour for the final six GPs interviewed.

Three GPs invited me to their homes—one for a weekend, and two for half-days—to facilitate discussion. Interviews became more akin to conversations in these more relaxed settings (a point noted by patients in their preference for home visits), and gave me a chance to recheck the data. At the end of each interview, I completed a brief Fact Sheet which provided basic sociodemographic details. I recorded some twenty hours of taped conversations which, when transcribed unedited, yielded some two hundred and fifty typed pages of material.

Unlike patients, only three GPs returned the transcripts with comments, and I decided to discontinue the exercise. However, the three GPs who did respond helped to confirm—and modify—my original interpretations. Further studies could usefully pursue this approach. Four GPs agreed to comment on earlier drafts of this book and some of their observations have been taken account of in the text. I asked Dr Quinn for permission to reproduce the very personal information he gave me, and he gladly agreed.

AND AFTER . . .

Transcription was time-consuming. It took one to one and a half days to type up an interview and I am not a slow typist. But it was richly rewarding. I was forced to go through the tapes in minute detail, sieving and categorizing both within and across transcripts in the continuous search for connections. This stimulated analysis.

The coding process enabled me to transform the veritable mountain of data into categories. Coding itself took a great deal of time. After each interview, I cut up and filed the transcript according to broad patterns of response, which were then tested, refined, and sometimes rejected as data collection proceeded. A similar exercise was then performed across transcripts. Coding was accompanied by simple numerical counting to confirm, or disconfirm, the direction of my findings, as Silverman (1985) suggests. I had folders of developing thoughts as ideas and concepts occurred and matured. As the research progressed, there was a continuous, cumulative interplay between ideas and data, between the particular and the general, from which the analytic framework of this book ultimately emerged.

STUDYING THE POWERLESS AND THE POWERFUL

I can now turn to the interlocking questions of involvement, responsibility and power, and their consequences for what emerged as data.

Enabling the Powerless: How Deep Should You Go?

I was in a privileged position with patients. I knew what living with chronic illness was like and yet had much to learn about the particular P.D. experience. But I was an insider. I did not need to manufacture a research role. It was tailor-made. In response to my explanation of why I was doing the study, Mrs Unwin remarked: 'You know what it's all about then.' Insider status had advantages and disadvantages. It allowed me to explore where others may not have been able to do so. At the same time, it was probably more difficult to maintain that delicate balance between overinvolvement and developing the kind of relationships which would facilitate the research process. Getting the balance right required constant monitoring.

I had to become involved if I was going to explore personal aspects of patients' lives. Moreover, I could not remain in people's houses for many hours over weeks and sometimes months and remain detached. Contact with patients was not restricted to interviews. I wanted to help where I could. This has involved me in letter-writing, sweeping snow, unblocking drains, preparing music for a Branch evening meeting, accompanying one patient to the theatre, another to the cinema—activities generally considered to break the rules of 'proper interviewing'. Not to have done them would have meant adopting a stance at variance with the spirit in which I conducted this research. Not only were they things I wanted to do; they were essential to the deeper understanding of the patients' experience of P.D.

Information—a Two-way Exchange
Such involvement raised questions both of power and of managing such emotional commitment. My aim was to empower patients. Sharing information was integral to this. In contrast to many research settings—including that in which I conducted some of the GP interviews—where it is the interviewer who asks the questions (Oakley, 1981), patients questioned me. They asked about my husband, how we 'coped', what kind of difficulties we had found and what our experience was with doctors. They also wanted to know how the research was going to be used and how it would help them. Some wanted information about the illness and the drug regimen. Others wondered about the other patients I had seen, how they compared physically and how they coped—intimate knowledge which membership of the Parkinson's Disease Society and attendance at local Branch meetings did not always necessarily provide. Patients were eager to reach out to others in the same predicament. They also asked questions about the GPs I had seen and about how my experiences agreed or disagreed with their own. Miss Evans, for example, wanted to know if other patients had been as lucky with their GPs as she had.

I answered personal questions with, I hope, the candour with which patients related their own experiences to me. In doing so, it made me rethink my own position on some issues. I discovered that I was more of a Weaver than I had thought. I answered questions about other patients and GPs in more general terms. In making any observations, scrupulous care was taken to ensure that nothing methodologically compromising—and, of course, nothing of a confidential nature—was revealed.

Questions about the research were also answered fully and frankly. Working over the transcripts with patients and revising drafts in the light of their comments made the research a collaborative venture. *Their* stories were going to be heard and it was our joint responsibility to get them right. As a result, my work had to be checked as well as theirs. Such consultation was not simply a validation exercise, although it was important that patients were able to recognize themselves in later analyses. It also formed another valuable source of data. Most importantly, as Mishler (1986) and

Cannon (1989) have recognized, the very process of consultation made the researcher–researched relationship much less one-sided—a point GPs may find helpful in thinking about the relationship between patient and doctor.

Other questions were less easy to answer. I had carefully tailored preceding talks to respect the wishes of Mr and Mrs Richards not to know the implications of having P.D., and was taken aback when, at a late stage in the interviews, Mrs Richards suddenly asked what the side-effects of the drugs were. I was both witness and, to an unknown extent, party to a radical shift in their perspective. In dealing honestly and responsibly with this situation, I began to appreciate something of the task facing GPs. I had the facts but was unsure how best to convey them. I concentrated on the side-effects I knew Mr Richards was experiencing at the time, checked the facts at home and gave the couple some references where they could pursue the question in more detail if they wished. The decision to give Mr and Mrs Mitchell a reference book posed similar dilemmas.

How Deep Can You Go?

Research with patients also raised emotional difficulties. Situations were often quite raw, particularly where spouses were involved. I could unwittingly disturb the delicate balance often negotiated between people to maintain a *modus vivendi*. For Mrs Jenson this was a welcome relief from tension: 'This is a wonderful excuse you being here for us to air things we probably wouldn't have discussed. . . . I'm glad you *can* disturb the balance, because there comes a time when one's literally boiling inside and not to have the outlet to say what one's thinking. . . .' I could not know of those occasions when my presence had less desirable outcomes. If this was the case, people did not say—or perhaps terminated the research process (one patient).

The situation of Mr and Mrs York was also distressing. I found Mrs York in bed, quite unable to carry on, crying aloud in despair—cries which were all too audible in the adjacent room, where her husband sat, wheelchair-bound and virtually speechless. I was depressed, helpless. An army of social workers and helpers had been unable to resolve the situation. As a carer myself, was this going to be me in ten years' time?

There were happier times, of course. Conversations were both enjoyable and sometimes hilarious. I have described the difficulties in order to make the more general point: I had underestimated the emotional demands working with P.D. patients would involve. I thought that I was sufficiently prepared, but found that this was not always the case. The Steering Group meetings which the Parkinson's Disease Society set up to exchange ideas about the development of the research were not forums where this kind of anxiety could be aired. I am not suggesting that researchers should be counsellors, but I was grateful for the counselling experience I had had in the past.

Research of this kind is not a responsibility to be undertaken lightly. Patients were intensely vulnerable. A wrong word here, a misplaced emphasis there, could quite unwittingly leave patients distressed and anxious. Precisely because of the heavy emotional commitment necessary, such research requires the ability to know where to stop. The periods when I could take time out to write up notes and reflect were often welcome respites. For this purpose, people had to be seen as data—a difficult but necessary distancing step.

In choosing to become involved and to empower patients in this way, the parameters were wide but were nonetheless there. Patients could choose how far they wanted to use them, and one or two preferred a more detached approach. But I set the rules, even though there were few rules. Unlike GPs, patients also had time. It was not that they did not have other commitments, particularly family ones. Managing the illness also often encroached on our time together. There was nothing I could do when patients had muscle spasms or experienced 'offs'. Conversation simply ceased. But I was the busy one. They filled time-slots in my diary, not vice versa. This was an imbalance I could never rectify. In that most patients responded very positively to this degree of commitment, I can only hope that it has enabled them to tell their stories in the way they wanted, and that the research experience has been as enriching for them as it has been for me—and, in turn, will enhance the reader's understanding.

Studying GPs: Equality of a Different Kind?

Interviewing the powerful as well as the powerless was a challenge. It raised sharply the question of 'whose side are we on?' (Becker, 1967). Traditionally, sociologists have concentrated on researching the powerless. Vulnerable groups in our society such as patients are much easier to approach, more amenable to lending their lives to investigation and less able to challenge the power of the researcher. They are the groups with whom many sociologists are happier to identify.

Interviewing those who hold positions of prestige and influence in our society, on the other hand, poses rather different questions. In this case, researching GPs had as much to do with mediating between patients and doctors as with addressing the imbalance of power between researcher and researched. Here I was engaged in a form of advocacy. I saw my task as one of translating the concerns patients had identified into issues for discussion with GPs.

Altering the Balance
Questions of involvement—ethical and emotional—were of a different order from those raised when talking with patients. I did not expect, nor was it appropriate for me to do so, to become involved with GPs in

anything like the depth which I have experienced with patients. Apart from the initial briefing, I said little—and was not asked much—about the research. The one personal detail I sometimes mentioned was my husband's M.S. This facilitated the making of comparisons and contrasts and was a valuable topic area in itself. However, only a few doctors tapped my experience of living with chronic illness. Others, whether from shyness, reticence or possibly unease, left it alone.

There was less demand for emotional input. I have shown the vital need for sensitivity in what was asked of, and said to, patients. Doctors were much less vulnerable. I did not have to worry about the possible effects of a slip of the tongue or a misplaced emphasis. Thus, as with patients, issues of involvement and power had important consequences for what emerged as accounts.

Researching GPs, too, was full of hopes, anxieties and expectations. It is fair to say that I approached the task of interviewing them with mixed feelings. I was an outsider. At the same time I was a peer, although my being a doctor (a PhD) but not a medic created some ambiguities. I learned later with astonishment, for instance, that Dr Victor had been 'very nervous' about being interviewed.

Changing Ideas

Despite my initial apprehensions, interviewing turned out to be a thoroughly pleasurable experience. It was apparent that GPs rarely had the chance to discuss their work with interested outsiders. For some it was enjoyable in itself and enabled them to appraise their ideas more critically. Dr Leadbrough said:

> It's a luxury to have someone listening. We spend so much time listening to others. It's very therapeutic. I actually feel better. I had flu last week and I feel better than I did this morning. . . . My non-medical student friends, they tend to want to know all the gory details, not about the work generally.

I appreciated the candour with which some GPs discussed their perceived shortcomings. Talks were often punctuated by remarks such as 'I know I fall down on that' or 'The more we talk the more I realize I don't say nearly enough'. Other GPs were also aware of the gap between their ideas and practice, as one GP commented: 'I'm aware that I'm not being strictly honest. I don't always do the things I'm saying.' The interviews thus gave GPs the chance to reflect on their work. Dr Threadgold commented afterwards: 'These aren't things you can give glib answers to. . . . You've set me thinking and given me things to think about. . . . It's quite a good experience to be on the receiving end of questions *you* want to ask.'

In many of the interviews, I experienced a genuine sense of warmth and interest. Direct contact gave me a chance to go back-stage and experience a little of what it was like being on the other side of the desk.

Many of my earlier ideas about doctors changed. I had never met a GP socially or as a 'colleague'. They were much less aloof and impersonal than I had expected. The confidence of judgement which my experience as a patient had led me to expect was much less evident. I was also surprised to discover the diffidence with which some GPs viewed academics. I had not thought of myself particularly as an 'ivory tower academic', having worked at grass-roots level for much of my life. The depth of even these comparatively short interviews enabled me to understand doctors in a way in which I had hitherto failed. They emerged for me as real people, with dilemmas and difficulties not so dissimilar from mine. It was a journey of discovery and an important antidote to the image of the doctor as powerful.

Some Problems

Interviews also had their difficulties, which sprung from the status of doctors as respected professionals. Apart from the three conducted in doctors' homes, the remainder were held in GPs' surgeries, and two in teaching hospitals. I was on their ground, not mine.

Time was a crucial issue. If I was to get anywhere, self-presentation had to be fast and to have immediate impact. As a highly valued commodity for GPs, time constrained what I was able to accomplish. I was a small slot in their busy diaries, someone to be fitted in rather than someone doing the fitting. As a sociologist a forty-five-minute interview was a short expenditure of time for me. It evidently represented a lot of time for GPs. I also wanted to respond to what was being said, to think ahead and put in a new question which had arisen. Sometimes this calls for reflection for a moment or two, but there was rarely time for reflection. I considered that I was not in a position to overrun. If GPs wanted to, that was a different matter, and my time was adjusted accordingly.

My hearing impairment turned out to be more of a handicap than I had imagined. I did not want to keep asking for repeats: as in most social interaction, it makes one appear stupid. Although I had hoped for some degree of accommodation—they were, after all, doctors—I found that the impairment was quickly forgotten. This meant straining to hear in some cases, which often added to the difficulty of conducting shorter interviews. I had to rely heavily on my tape recorder for picking up missed pieces, but even so, occasional phrases and passages were lost.

Finally, for ten GPs these were one-off interviews, unlike my talks with patients. I was unable to return to clarify any misunderstandings or ambiguities, which often only emerged in typing the transcript. My understanding was immeasurably enriched for those five GPs with whom I later corresponded and talked.

Researching doctors was not comparable to studying patients in terms of its involvement and its impact on both my life and theirs. Yet my sympathies were engaged. I was able to understand something of the difficulties of GPs facing patients with a chronic illness which a survey approach could never have revealed—an understanding I believe readers will share.

....

I hope that by placing patients' and GPs' stories in a wider framework, this may enable them to see their own positions in a different light. Ultimately the merits of such an approach depend on the fidelity and integrity with which I have captured the meanings of what patients and GPs said. The book will have succeeded in its task if I, as privileged researcher and participant, have been able to convey to readers something of the flavour and richness of what patients and GPs experience in the course of trying to manage P.D. It is their stories which ask to be heard.

Appendix 1: Patient Profile

Patient	Age	Age at confirmation of diagnosis	Duration of illness at time of interview	Family status	Occupational status
Mr Canning	59	59	1 year	Lives at home with wife	Headmaster (retired)
Mr Mitchell	62	60	2 years	Lived with disabled wife. Died December 1986	Signalman (early retirement on health grounds)
Mr Richards	72	69	2½ years	Lived with wife and family. Died January 1987	Teacher (retired)
Mr York	75	71	c. 4 years	Lived with wife. Transferred to nursing home 1987	Freelance photographer (retired)
Mrs Pembridge	61	57	4 years	Lives alone. Separated from husband. Transferred to sheltered accommodation 1987	Secretary/book-keeper. Not worked for several years
Mr Jenson	65	60	5½ years	Lived with wife (retired clerical officer). Died April 1988	Project engineer (retired)
Mrs Franklin	54	47	7 years	Lives with husband (both working)	Estate agent/negotiator

Patient	Age	Age at confirmation of diagnosis	Duration of illness at time of interview	Family status	Occupational status
Miss Evans	66	59	7 years	Lives in sheltered accommodation	State Registered Nurse/typist (retired)
Mr Grenville	43	35	7½ years	Lives with wife (works as teacher) and family	Lecturer
Mrs Quentin	74	63	10 years	Lived alone in sheltered accommodation. Died September 1987	Welfare officer (retired)
Mr Unwin	74	64	11 years	Lives with wife. Moved to sheltered accommodation 1985	Tyre-builder (retired)
Mr Irving	63	51	12 years	Lived with wife at home. Wife died 1988. Transferred to nursing home	Professional association officer (retired)
Mr Vernon	61	49	12 years	Lives with wife (retired Health Visitor) at home	Sales representative (early retirement with P.D.)
Mr Dempsey	55	44	12 years	Widower. Lives alone	Plumber (early retirement with P.D.)
Miss Norton	60	35	25 years	Lived alone. Married 1987	Ward clerk (not worked for many years)

Appendix 2: Doctor Profile

Doctor	Age	Gender	Years in practice
Dr Black	29	Male	2
Dr Dandridge	65	Female	33
Dr Smythe	30	Male	4
Dr Fleming	30	Male	$2\frac{1}{2}$
Dr Naughton	35	Male	$6\frac{1}{2}$
Dr Victor	57	Male	29
Dr Perlmann	33	Male	3
Dr Miller	39	Female	6
Dr Wilkinson	40	Male	8
Dr Arlen	57	Female	25
Dr Richards	30	Male	3
Dr Quinn	66	Male	30 (retired 1985; does locums)
Dr Young	34	Female	$4\frac{1}{2}$
Dr Ogilvie	30	Male	Trainee
Dr Clements	45	Female	*c*. 20
Dr Threadgold	39	Male	13
Dr Ellis	54	Female	16
Dr Leadbrough	39	Female	5

References

Alexander, L. (1980). The double-bind between dialysis patients and their health practitioners. In Eisenberg, L. and Kleinman, A. (Eds), *The Relevance of Social Science for Medicine*. D. Reidel, Dordrecht

Anderson, R. and Bury, M. (Eds) (1988). *Living with Chronic Illness: The Experience of Patients and Their Families*. Unwin Hyman, London

Arluke, A. (1980). Judging drugs: patients' conceptions of therapeutic efficacy in the treatment of arthritis. *Human Organization*, **39** (1), 84–87

Atkinson, P. (1984). Training for certainty. *Soc. Sci. Med.*, **19** (9), 949–956

Baker, M. G. and Pinder, M. R. (1989). Relations between the disabled and chronic sick and society: towards a better understanding. *Int. J. Adv. Counselling*, **12**, 137–142

Barbeau, A. (1981). The L-dopa story 1958–1979. In Clifford-Rose, F. and Capildeo, R. (Eds), *Research Progress in Parkinson's Disease*. Pitman, London

Barnlund, D. C. (1976). The mystification of meaning: doctor–patient encounters. *J. Med. Educ.*, **57**, 716–725

Baruch, G. (1981). Moral tales: parents' stories of encounters with the health professionals. *Soc. Hlth Illness*, **3** (3), 275–295

de Beauvoir, S. (1970). *Old Age*. Penguin, Harmondsworth

Becker, H. S. (1967). Whose side are we on? *Soc. Problems*, **14**, 239–247

Berg, D. (1988). Anxiety in research relationships. In Berg, D. B. and Smith, K. K. (Eds), *The Self in Social Inquiry: Researching Methods*. Sage Publications, California and London

Blumhagen, D. (1980). Hyper-tension, a folk illness with a medical name. *Cult. Med. Psychiat.*, **4**, 197–227

Brocklehurst, J. C., Morris, P., Andrews, K., Richards, B. and Laycock, P. (1981). Social effects of stroke. *Soc. Sci. Med.*, **15A**, 35–39

Brownlea, A. (1987). Participation: myths, realities and prognosis. *Soc. Sci. Med.*, **25** (6), 605–614

Bury, M. (1982). Chronic illness as biographical disruption. *Soc. Hlth Illness*, **4** (2), 167–182

Bury, M. (1985). Dilemmas facing patients and providers in disablement. *Int. Rehab. Med.*, **7**, 162–166

Byrne, P. S. and Long, B. E. L. (1984). *Doctors Talking to Patients: A Study of the Verbal Behaviour of General Practitioners Consulting in their Surgeries*. Royal College of General Practitioners, London

Calnan, M. (1984). Clinical uncertainty: is it a problem in the doctor–patient relationship? *Soc. Hlth Illness*, **6** (1), 74–85

Cannon, S. (1989). Social research in stressful settings: difficulties for the sociologist studying the treatment of breast cancer. *Soc. Hlth Illness*, **11** (1), 62–77

Cantley, C. and Hunter, D. (1985). People processing: towards a typology of selected general practitioner referral and admission practices in the care of elderly people. *Ageing Soc.*, **5**, 267–288

Charmaz, K. (1983). Loss of self: a fundamental form of suffering in the chronically ill. *Soc. Hlth Illness*, **5** (2), 168–195

Cobb, A. K. and Hamera, E. (1986). Illness experience in a chronic disease—ALS. *Soc. Sci. Med.*, **23** (7), 641–650

Comaroff, J. (1976). Communicating information about non-fatal illness: the strategies of a group of general practitioners. *Soc. Rev.*, **24**, 269–287

Comaroff, J. and Maguire, P. (1981). Ambiguity and the search for meaning: childhood leukaemia in the modern clinical context. *Soc. Sci. Med.*, **15B**, 115–123

Darling, R. J. (1979). *Families against Society: A Study of Reactions to Children with Birth Defects*. Sage Publications, Newbury Park, Calif.

Davis, F. (1960). Uncertainty in medical prognosis clinical and functional. *Am. J. Soc.*, **66**, 41–47

Davis, F. (1963). *Passage through Crisis: Polio Victims and Their Families*. Bobbs-Merrill, New York

Dowd, J. (1975). Aging as exchange: a preface to theory. *J. Gerontol.*, **30** (5), 584–594

Dowie, R. (1983). *General Practitioners and Consultants: A Study of Outpatient Referrals*. King Edward's Hospital Fund, London

Duvoisin, R. (1984) *Parkinson's Disease: A Guide for Patient and Family*, 2nd edn. Raven Press, New York

Essex, L. (1983). One patient's view of Parkinson's Disease. *J. Roy. Soc. Hlth*, **5**, 169–173

Fennell, G., Phillipson, C. and Evers, H. (1988). *The Sociology of Old Age*. Open University Press, Milton Keynes

Fitzpatrick, R. and Hopkins, A. (1983). Problems in the conceptual framework of patient satisfaction research: an empirical exploration. *Soc. Hlth Illness*, **5** (3), 297–311

Fox, R. C. (1957). Training for uncertainty. In Cox, C. and Mead, A. (Eds), *A Sociology of Medical Practice*. Collier-Macmillan, London

Fox, R. C. (1959). *Experiment Perilous: Physicians and Patients Facing the Unknown*. Free Press, Glencoe

Fox, R. C. (1980). The evolution of medical uncertainty. *Milbank Memorial Fund Q.*, *Hlth Soc.*, **58** (1), 1–49

Freer, C. (1988). Old myths: frequent misconceptions about the elderly. In Wells, N. and Freer, C. (Eds), *The Ageing Population: Burden or Challenge?* Macmillan Press, Basingstoke

Gerson, E. M. and Strauss, A. (1975). Time for living: problems in chronic illness care. *Soc. Policy*, Nov./Dec., 12–18

Godwin-Austen, R. B. (1984). *The Parkinson's Disease Handbook*. Sheldon Press, London

Godwin-Austen, R. B. and Hildick-Smith, M. (1982). *Parkinson's Disease: The General Practitioner's Guide*. Franklin Scientific Projects, London

Goffman, E. (1963). *Stigma: Notes on the Management of Spoiled Identity*. Prentice-Hall, Englewood Cliffs, New Jersey

Hasler, J. C. (1985). The very stuff of general practice. *J. Roy. Coll. Gen. Pract.*, **35**, 121–127

Hauser, S. T. (1981). Physician–patient relationships. In Mishler, E. G., Amarasingham, L. R., Hauser, S. T., Liem, R., Osherson, S. D. and Waxler, N. (Eds), *Social Contexts of Health, Illness and Patient Care*. Cambridge University Press, Cambridge

Hazan, H. (1980). *The Limbo People: A Study of the Constitution of the Time Universe among the Aged*. Routledge and Kegan Paul, London

Helman, C. (1984). *Culture, Health and Illness*. John Wright, Bristol

Hildick-Smith, M. (1980). Management of Parkinson's Disease in the elderly. In Denham, M. D. (Ed.), *The Treatment of Medical Problems in the Elderly*. MTP Press, Lancaster

Horobin, G. (1983). Professional mystery: the maintenance of charisma in general practice. In Dingwall, R. and Lewis, P. (Eds), *The Sociology of the Professions: Lawyers, Doctors and Others*. Macmillan Press, Basingstoke

Jefferys, M. and Sachs, H. (1983). *Rethinking General Practice: Dilemmas in Primary Medical Care*. Tavistock, London

Jobling, R. (1988). The experience of psoriasis under treatment. In Anderson, R. and Bury, M. (Eds), *Living with Chronic Illness: The Experience of Patients and Their Families*. Unwin Hyman, London

Jobling, R. G. and Coles, R. B. (1988). The skin patient: the need for information. *Dermatol. Pract.*, June, 6–7

Kelleher, D. (1988). *Diabetes*. Routledge, London

Kelly, M. (1987). Adjusting to ileostomy. *Nursing Times*, **83** (33), 29–31

Kleinman, A. (1988). *The Illness Narratives: Suffering, Healing and the Human Condition*. Basic Books, New York

Knafl, K. and Burkett, G. (1978). Professional socialization in a surgical speciality: acquiring medical judgement. In Schwartz, H. D. and Kart, C. S. (Eds), *Dominant Issues in Medical Sociology*. Addison-Wesley, Reading, Mass.

Light, D. (1979). Uncertainty and control in professional training. *J. Hlth Soc. Behav.*, **20** (Dec.), 310–322

Locker, D. (1983). *Disability and Disadvantage: The Consequences of Chronic Illness*. Tavistock, London

Locker, D. and Dunt, D. (1978). Theoretical and methodological issues in sociological studies of consumer satisfaction with medical care. *Soc. Sci. Med.*, **12**, 283–292

Locker, D. and Kaufert, J. (1988). The breath of life: medical technology and the careers of people with post-respiratory poliomyelitis. *Soc. Hlth Illness*, **10** (1), 23–40

McIntosh, J. (1977). *Communication and Awareness in a Cancer Ward*. Croom Helm, London

Maguire, P. (1984). Communication skills and patient care. In Steptoe, A. and Mathews, A. (Eds), *Health Care and Human Behaviour*. Academic Press, London

Maguire, P. (1985). Barriers to the psychological care of the dying. *Br. Med. J.*, **291**, 1711–1713

Maguire, P., Fairburn, S. and Fletcher, C. (1986). Consulting skills of young doctors. *Br. Med. J.*, **292**, 1573–1576

Maguire, P. and Faulkner, A. (1988). Improve the counselling skills of doctors and nurses in cancer care. *Br. Med. J.*, **297**, 847–849

Marsden, C. D. and Parkes, J. D. (1976). 'On–off' effects in patients with Parkinson's Disease on chronic levodopa therapy. *Lancet*, **1**, 292–296

Marsden, C. D., Parkes, J. D. and Quinn, N. (1982). Fluctuations of disability in Parkinson's Disease—clinical aspects. In Marsden, C. D. and Fahn, S. (Eds), *Movement Disorders*. Butterworths, Borough Green, Kent

Mason, C. (1985). The production and effects of uncertainty with special reference to diabetes mellitus. *Soc. Sci. Med.*, **21** (12), 1329–1334

Mishler, E. G. (1986). *Research Interviewing: Context and Narrative*. Harvard University Press, Cambridge, Mass.

Morgan, J. (1988). Living with renal failure on home haemodyalisis. In Anderson, R. and Bury, M. (Eds), *Living with Chronic Illness: The Experience of Patients and Their Families*. Unwin Hyman, London

Morgan, M., Calnan, M. and Manning, N. (1985). *Sociological Approaches to Health and Medicine*. Croom Helm, London

Murphy, R. F. (1987). *The Body Silent*. Dent, London

Mutch, W. J., Dingwall-Fordyce, I., Downie, A. W., Paterson, J. G. and Roy, S. K. (1986). Parkinson's Disease in a Scottish city. *Br. Med. J.*, **292**, 534–536

Oakley, A. (1981). Interviewing women—a contradiction in terms. In Roberts, H. (Ed.), *Doing Feminist Research*. Routledge and Kegan Paul, London

Office of Health Economics (1974). *Parkinson's Disease*. Studies of Current Health Problems, Number 51. Office of Health Economics, London

Oliver, M., Zarb, G., Silver, J., Moore, M. and Salisbury, V. (1988). *Walking into Darkness: The Experience of Spinal Cord Injury*. Macmillan Press, Basingstoke

O.P.C.S. Monitor (1986). Population projections: mid-1985-based. 16 Dec., PP2 86/1

Parkinson, J. (1817). *An Essay on the Shaking Palsy*. Sherwood, Neely and Jones, London

The Parkinson Study Group (1989). Effects of deprenyl on the progression of disability in early Parkinson's disease. *New Engl. J. Med.*, **321**, 1364–1371

Pearlin, L. T. and Schooler, C. (1978). The structure of coping. *J. Hlth Soc. Behav.*, **19**, 2–21

Pendleton, D. and Hasler, J. (1983). Doctor–patient communication: a review. In Pendleton, D. and Hasler, J. (Eds), *Doctor–Patient Communication*. Academic Press, London

Pinder, M. R. (1983). Stigma, Stereotyping and Strategy Management of the Adult Hearing Impaired at Work. PhD Thesis, Brunel University, Uxbridge

Pinder, M. R. (1988). Striking balances: living with Parkinson's Disease. In Anderson, R. and Bury, M. (Eds), *Living with Chronic Illness: The Experience of Patients and Their Families*. Unwin Hyman, London

Posner, T. (1977). Magical elements in orthodox medicine: diabetes as a medical thought system. In Dingwall, R., Heath, C., Reid, M. and Stacey, M. (Eds), *Health Care and Health Knowledge*. Croom Helm, London

Posner, T. (1988). Sailing single-handed: autonomy in the control of diabetes. *Int. Disability Studies*, **10** (3), 123–128

Power, P. W. and Sax, D. S. (1978). The communication of information to the neurological patient: some implications for family coping. *J. Chron. Dis.*, **31**, 57–65

Prottas, J. M. (1979). *People Processing: The Street Level Bureaucrat in Public Service Bureaucracies*. Lexington Books, Lexington, Mass.

Quine, L. and Pahl, J. (1986). First diagnosis of severe mental handicap: characteristics of unsatisfactory encounters between doctors and patients. *Soc. Sci. Med.*, **15B**, 115–123

Ridsdale, L. (1987). Communicating with our patients: helping the helpers. *Practitioner*, **231**, 1167–1168

Roberts, H. (1985). *The Patient Patients: Women and Their Doctors*. Pandora Press, London

Robinson, I. (1988). *Multiple Sclerosis*. Routledge, London

Rosser, V. E. and Maguire, P. (1982). Dilemmas in general practice: the care of the cancer patient. *Soc. Sci. Med.*, **16**, 315–322

Roth, J. (1963). *Timetables: Structuring the Passage of Time in Hospital Treatment and Other Careers*. Bobbs-Merrill, New York

Royal College of Physicians (1986). Physical disability in 1986 and beyond. *J. Roy. Coll. Phys.*, **20** (3), 160–194

Sanson-Fisher, R. and Maguire, P. (1980). Should skills in communicating with patients be taught in medical schools? *Lancet*, **2**, 523–526

Schneider, J. W. and Conrad, P. (1983). *Having Epilepsy: The Experience and Control of Illness*. Temple University Press, Philadelphia

Schoenberg, B. S. (1986). Descriptive epidemiology of Parkinson's Disease: disease distribution and hypothesis formulation. *Adv. Neurol.*, **45**, 277–283

Silverman, D. (1985). *Qualitative Methodology and Sociology: Describing the Social World*. Gower Publishing, Aldershot

Speedling, E. J. (1982). *Heart Attack: The Family Response at Home and in the Hospital*. Tavistock, London

Stern, G. and Lees, A. (1982). *Parkinson's Disease: The Facts*. Oxford University Press, Oxford

Stibe, C. M. H., Lees, A. J., Kempster, P. A. and Stern, G. M. (1988). Subcutaneous apomorphine in Parkinsonian on–off oscillations. *Lancet*, **1**, 403–406

Still, A. W. and Todd, C. J. (1986). Role ambiguity in general practice: the care of patients dying at home. *Soc. Sci. Med.*, **23** (5), 519–525

Strauss, A., Fagerhaugh, S., Suczek, B. and Wiener, C. (1985). *Social Organization of Medical Work*. University of Chicago Press, Chicago

Strauss, A. and Glaser, B. (Eds) (1975). *Chronic Illness and the Quality of Life*. Mosby, St. Louis

Taylor, K. M. (1988). 'Telling bad news': physicians and the disclosure of undesirable information, *Soc. Hlth Illness*, **10** (2), 109–132

Thompson, J. (1984). Communicating with patients. In Fitzpatrick, R., Hinton, J., Newman, S., Scambler, G. and Thompson, J. (Eds), *The Experience of Illness*. Tavistock, London

Thompson, M. K. (1987). *Caring for Your Parkinsonian Patients*. Royal College of General Practitioners, London

Tuckett, D., Boulton, M., Olson, C. and Williams, A. (1985). *Meetings between Experts: An Approach to Sharing Ideas in Medical Consultations*. Tavistock, London

Update (1984). Parkinson's Disease. 15 Aug., 256–261

Verby, J. E., Holden, P. and Davis, R. H. (1979). Peer review of consultations in primary care: the use of audiovisual recordings. *Br. Med. J.*, **1**, 1686–1688

Victor, C. R. (1987). *Old Age in Modern Society: A Textbook of Social Gerontology*. Croom Helm, London

Waddell, C. (1982). The process of neutralisation and the uncertainties of cystic fibrosis. *Soc. Hlth Illness*, **4**, 210–220

Wadel, C. (1979). The hidden work of everyday life. In Wallman, S. (Ed.), *Social Anthropology of Work*. Academic Press, London

Walker, M. (1988). Training the trainers: socialisation and change in general practice. *Soc. Hlth Illness*, **10** (3), 282–302

West, P. (1976). The physician and the management of childhood epilepsy. In Wadsworth, M. and Robinson, D. (Eds), *Studies in Everyday Medical Life*. Martin Robertson, London

Weston, W. W. and Lipkin, M. (1989). Doctors learning communication skills: developmental issues. In Stewart, M. and Roter, D. (Eds), *Communicating with Medical Patients*. Sage Publications, Newbury Park, Calif.

Wiener, C. (1975). The burden of rheumatoid arthritis: tolerating the uncertainty. *Soc. Sci. Med.*, **9**, 97–104

Wiener, C., Fagerhaugh, S., Strauss, A. and Suczek, B. (1980). Patient power: complex issues need complex answers. *Soc. Policy*, Sept./Oct., 30–37

Williams, G. H. and Wood, P. H. N. (1986). Common-sense beliefs about illness: a mediating role for the doctor. *Lancet*, **2**, 1435–1437

Williams, G. H. and Wood, P. H. N. (1988). Coming to terms with chronic illness: the negotiation of autonomy in rheumatoid arthritis. *Int. Disability Studies*, **10** (3), 128–133

Wilmer, H. A. (1987). The doctor–patient relationship and the issues of pity, sympathy and empathy. In Stoeckle, J. (Ed.), *Encounters between Patients and Doctors: An Anthology*. M.I.T. Press, Cambridge, Mass.

Wilson, J. A. (1986). Management of Parkinson's Disease in general practice. *Scott. Med. J.*, **31**, 132–134

Wynne, A. (1988). Accounting for accounts in Multiple Sclerosis. In Woolgar, S. (Ed.), *Knowledge and Reflexivity: New Frontiers in the Sociology of Knowledge*. Sage Publications, California and London

Zola, I. (1983). *Socio-Medical Inquiries: Recollections, Reflections, and Reconsiderations*. Temple University Press, Philadelphia

Index

Abilities, loss of 85
Aborted fetuses 10
Accounts, different, patients' and
    GPs' 3, 115
Activities, loss of 85
Acute illnesses
    care rather than cure 107
    dichotomy between 68-71
    and dichotomy between acute versus
        chronic illnesses 106
Age 13
    judgements concerning 19, 23, 50,
        104
Ageism 12
AIDS 59
Amitryptyline 64
Anonymity
    preservation of 8
    see also Research methodology and
        method
Anticholinergic drugs 9, 44
Anxiety 23, 41, 44, 46-47, 66-67, 72,
    74, 77
    accompanying Parkinson's disease 5
    after failure of drug regimens to live
        up to expectations 55
    arousal of 22
    of GPs 3, 68, 70
    GPs' explorations of patients' 71-75
    manifested openly by GPs to patients'
        own distress 80
    new sources of 54
    as new symptoms develop 89
    prevarication in relation to 29
    settling of 28-29
    see also under Discomfort; Distress;
        Fear; Uncertainty; Unease
Avoiders 52, 55, 66

and anxiety 26, 31-34

Beliefs 11-24
    adoption of 52-53
    of GPs
        and explanations in relation to
            patients' ages 12, 23-24
        and explanations in relation to
            patients' educational
            backgrounds 12, 23-24
        and explanations in relation to
            patients' intelligence 12, 23-24
        and explanations in relation to
            what patients can cope with 17,
            23-25
Breast cancer 15, 74
Bromocriptine 9

Cancer 100
Cancer patients 5, 68, 73
    communication with 6
    Seekers 26
Care, pastoral 80
Care rather than cure 107
Chronic illnesses xii, 1, 62-63, 68-70,
    76-77, 80-81, 85-86, 89, 94,
    96-97, 99-101, 108-111, 115,
    120, 123, 125
    management of xi, 5, 103
    and patient-doctor relationships 2
    psychological and social sequelae
        of 94, 101
    studies of 5-6, 106
Clinical decision-making, sharing of
    patients in 50-52
Clinical uncertainty 6
    deliberate emphasis of 19-20

Communication
  patient-doctor   xi-xii, 4
  see also Uncertainty, management of;
    Patient-doctor relationships
Communication and speech
    deterioration   70-71
Communication strategies   16-17
  see also Uncertainty, management of
Conditions for change   98-99
Confidentiality   121
Counselling   14, 74, 110
  groups for   79, 81
  need for, *see* Recommendations for
    future practice
Cystic fibrosis   6

Day centres   115
Decarboxylase inhibitors
  Madopar   9
  Sinemet   9
Decision-making problems   24, 41-53,
    68-82
Dependence   64, 83, 90, 101, 106, 108
  wheelchairs as a focus for   84
Deprenyl   9-10
Depression   64, 91-93, 96, 107
Dermatitis
  seborrhoeic   55
  see also Drugs, side-effects of
Detachment, *see under* GPs
Diabetes   xi, 6, 50-51, 54, 60, 100
  drug regimens in   48
Diagnoses   4, 6, 11, 15, 31, 55, 103-
    104, 109
  difficulties in   2
  and new uncertainties   25
  and Seekers   26
Disabilities
  and age   13
  communication   71
  facial expression   70
  hearing   71
  memory impairment   70
  speech deterioration   9, 70
Discomfort   79
Distress   3, 63, 72-74, 77-81, 108
  causing   2
  counselling approach to   24
  in managing drug regimens   54
Dixarit   64
Doctor profiles   7, 128
Doctor-patient relationships, *see*

  Patient-doctor relationships
Dopamine   9-10
Drug dependency, fear of   58, 106
Drug management
  'honeymoon period'   10, 54-67
  see also under GPs, strategies to
    manage uncertainty/anxiety
Drug regimens   7, 41-53, 95, 97, 103,
    106, 121
  limitations of   41-67
  multiple   56
  rationale of   41-44
  side-effects of   44-48, 59, 66, 105,
    107
  and treatments   xi, 41-53
  unease about   43
  unpredictability of   57-59
Drugs
  antidepressant   64
  dependency on   57-59, 67
  medical complacency in relation
    to   57-59
  non-compliance   43
  other   58, 64
  overdoses, risk of   49, 53, 60
  side-effects of
    involuntary writhing
      movements   9
    'on-off' syndrome   10, 49
    seborrhoeic dermatitis   55

Education
  medical   109
  see also Training and medical
    education
Emotional stability, judgements
    about   17-19, 45, 104
Emotional support, provision of   6, 68-
    82
Epilepsy   47, 54
  drug treatment in   42
Euthanasia   93
Explanations   11-24
  by doctors to patients   11-24
  and age   12-15
  ambiguity in   12
  and beliefs and routines   11-24
  and educational attainment   15-17
  and emotional stability   17, 19, 23,
    45, 104
  flexibility in   12
  frankness in   12

and intelligence of patients 15, 17,
23, 104
open and closed policies
towards 25-39

Facial expression 70
Fact sheets 117, 119
Fear
causing of 2
of drug dependency 58
GPs' explorations of 71-75
patients' responses to 83-96
Fetal transplants 7
Flexibility in GPs' attitudes 8, 24, 73,
100
towards drug management 41-53
towards empathy 68-81
towards information giving 14
Frustration 3, 67
causing of, in patients 17
events leading to, in GPs 69-71, 79-
80
management of, *see* GPs, strategies
to manage uncertainty/anxiety
see also under Anxiety, causing of;
Uncertainty
Functional uncertainty 6

GP profiles 7, 128
GPs
access to 94, 118-119
anxieties of 3, 15
beliefs of 32, 41, 53
closed versus open approach of 8,
11-23, 41-53, 68-81, 97-109
empathy of 68-82
feelings of
helplessness and inadequacy 3,
68-81
'non-activity', discomfort
with 68-81
frustrations of 15
and implications for
communication xi, 3, 23, 53,
81, 97-111
involvement, managing the degree
of 69-82, 107
patients' views of 34-38, 63-66, 91-
95
policies of, towards patients 8, 11-
23, 41-53, 68-81, 97-109
roles of 34-38

selection criteria for, in
research 118
and strategies to manage uncertainty/
anxiety
counselling groups, help from 79
detachment/empathy, striking
balance between 68-81
functional uncertainty, use of 44
innovations, use of 19-23
judgements
use of
and beliefs about age,
intelligence, what patients
can cope with 12-19, 23-
24, 42-46, 52-53, 103-105
and emotional stability 17-
19, 45, 104
medical management/control of
drug regimens 49-50, 105
optimism, use of 19-21, 23, 47
question initiating and
responding 21-23
questions, use of 21-23
rescheduling, pacing 69, 72-74,
76, 81
restructuring own time 72-73, 81
restructuring patients' time
priorities 45, 47
focus on the present 45, 52
routines, use of 3, 19-23, 32, 41,
53
shared management of drugs 50-
52, 105
stressing variability of
prognosis 19
time, spinning out of 20, 69
and uncertainties 3

'Hidden work' 87
Hospital system, getting lost in 36-37,
92
'House style', GPs' use of 23, 104
Hypertension 77
drug treatment in 42

Identities
maintenance of 84-86, 88, 107
patients' preservation of 90, 95
Illiterate patients, judgements
about 16
Illness
acute 68-71

Illness – *continued*
  chronic, *see under* Chronic illnesses
  terminal   68-71
Implications
  of having Parkinson's disease
    coming to understand   25-40
    disclosure of   11-24
Incurability   9, 69-71
Independence, retention of   86
Individualized care   14, 39, 67, 100
  see also Patient as a person
Information
  acquisition of   25-40
  anxiety provoking nature of   42
  control of, and equivocation   29
  conveying of   6, 8, 15
  see also Knowledge and
    understanding, gap between
Innovations   19-23
  see also GPs, strategies to manage
    uncertainty/anxiety
Insulin   50-51
Intelligence of patients
  and judgements about   15-17, 104
  see also Explanations, and beliefs and
    routines
Intelligent patients, preferences
    for   15-17, 104
Interviews   117, 120, 123-125
  guide for   117
  multiple in-depth   7
  semistructured   113
Involvement
  determining degree of   69-82, 107
  see also under GPs, strategies to
    manage uncertainty and anxiety

'Joint partnerships'   35, 51-53, 65-66,
    109
  see also Shared decision-making
'Just being there'   75-80

Knowledge
  as a resource   25-40
  right Inoti to know   18
  and understanding, gap
    between   15, 24, 103-105

Levodopa therapy   9, 43, 49-51, 55,
    58-59, 65
Listening, difficulties of   75-80
Literate patients, judgements
    about   15

Loss, feelings of   2, 84-85
'Loss of self'   89

Madopar   9, 44
Marital strain   85-86, 101
Match and mismatch of perspectives,
    between patients and GPs   97-
    111
Matching question   113-115
Medical education   109-111
Medical management of drugs   48-52
  doctors supporting   49-50
Medical technology, haemodialysis   60
Memory disturbances   9
  see also Parkinson's disease, clinical
    features and symptoms of
Memory impairment   70
  see also Parkinson's disease, clinical
    features and symptoms of
Migraine   56, 64
  medication for, *see* Dixarit
Miscommunication   3
Misdiagnoses   9
Misunderstandings, in relation to
    treatment   55
Multiple sclerosis   x, 12, 17, 30, 46,
    100, 114, 123
Muscle spasms   90, 123

Nervous system, degenerative diseases
    of   8
'Non-activity', discomfort with   78-79
Non-compliance   43

Openness   14, 24
Optimism as a routine   19
  and the sparing of distress and
    anxiety   20-21
  use of   19-21
  see also GPs, strategies to manage
    uncertainty/anxiety
Osteoarthritis   76
Over-optimism, risks of   21

Pacing strategies   69, 72, 81
  see also GPs, strategies to manage
    uncertainty/anxiety
Parkinson's disease   x, 12, 14, 41, 113
  age of patients with   9, 52
  classical triad of symptoms in   8-9,
    28, 56, 59, 70-72, 86-87, 89-90,
    122
  clinical features and symptoms of   9,

28, 56, 59, 70-72, 86-87, 89-90, 122
  desire to be appraised of   28
  early symptoms   7-8
  episodes of freezing   9
  episodes of start-hesitation   9
  facial expression   70
  giddy turns   9
  impaired speech   8
  long term   9
  mood swings, unpredictable   9, 91
  muscle cramps   28
  muscle spasms   90, 123
  physical   87
  stooping gait in   9
  shuffling   86
  tremor   59
clinical uncertainty in   6, 9, 44, 51
diagnoses of   2, 4, 8-9, 11, 25, 27-28, 31, 36, 38, 55, 103-104
drug therapy and treatment in, and side-effects of   9-10, 41, 44-45, 47, 49, 52, 59, 66, 105, 121
early symptoms in   8-9
facts and figures on   8-10
fatigue   8
GPs' and patients' strategies in   83-96
  making a pact with   89-90
  making sense of living with   83-96
  search for control of   86-89
prognoses of   2-4, 6-23, 25, 28, 30, 32-33, 39, 69-71, 87, 98
in relation to other conditions   xii-xiii, 17, 30, 35, 42, 46-47, 50, 54, 56, 59-60, 68, 71, 73-74, 78, 100, 123
Parkinson's Disease Society   xi-xii, 87-88, 99, 111, 115, 119, 121-22
'Parkinson's face', and communication difficulties   69-71
Pastoral care   68-82
  role of GPs in   92-93
Patient as expert   105-106
Patient group, characteristics of   115-116
Patient as a person   40, 94, 109
Patient profiles   7, 126-127
Patient-doctor relationships
  and being on drugs, feelings about   57-59
  match and mismatch in perspectives in   103-109

strategies in
  accepting   83-96
  attempts at control   83-96
  'denial'   30, 90
  distancing   33, 88
  expertise, development of   54-67, 106
  fighting   86-87
  fundamental concerns of   83-96
  referents, use of   87-88
  restructuring of time perspectives   88-89
  routines, use of   3, 87, 89-90
  'switching off'   30-31
  timing and scheduling strategies   60-62
  see also Avoiders; Seekers; Weavers
Patients
  as partners with GPs   107, 109
    see also 'Joint partnerships'; Shared decision-making
  person-behind-patient   93, 95, 97-111
    see also Individualized care
    see also Anxiety; Distress; Fear
PD, *see* Parkinson's disease
'PD face', *see* Communication and speech deterioration; Parkinson's face, and communication difficulties
Poliomyelitis   6, 60
Powerless and powerful, studies of   120-125
Prognoses   6, 11, 22-23, 98
  doctors' strategies in stressing the variability of   19, 31
  patients' use of variability in   30-34
  see also Parkinson's disease
Progression   69-71
Psoriasis   54

Qualitative approaches   7, 113
Qualitative and quantitative research, relative merits of   112-125

Recommendations for future practice   109-111
Referents, use of   87-88
Renal failure   54
Replacement therapy, drug treatment as   9
Research issues   123

Research issues – *continued*
  involvement   113
  power   113
  responsibility   113
Research methodology and method   7-8, 112-125
  and chronic illness   112-125
Rheumatoid arthritis   xi, 6, 30
  drug treatment in   42
  see also under Drug regimens; Drugs
Rigidity symptoms   8
Routines   11-24, 89-90, 95, 98
  adoption of   52-53
  development of
    by GPs   12
    by patients and GPs   3
    see also under GPs, strategies to
    manage uncertainty/anxiety;
    Patient-doctor relationships,
    routine use of
  as a means of holding negative
    feelings in check   87
  and the use of optimism   19-21

Stooping gait   9
Scheduling strategies   114
Seekers   26-28, 52, 56-57, 66
  see also Information, control of, and
    equivocation
Selection criteria, for research
    subjects   113, 115, 118
Selegiline   9
Self-determination   87
Shared decision-making, *see* 'Joint
    partnerships'
Shared management of drugs and
    illness   48-53
  doctors supporting   50-52
  see also Drug management; 'Joint
    partnerships'
Side-effects   9-10, 49, 52, 56-57, 59, 66,
    121
  see also Drug regimens; Drugs
Sinemet   9, 42-43
Social class   116
  judgements about   16
  of patients   16
Social isolation   85
Speech
  and communication difficulties   70
  comprehensibility of   30-31, 70-71
  deterioration in clarity and volume
    of   9, 70

Start hesitation   9
Stereotactic surgery   65
Stereotypes   13
  about age   23
Strategies, *see under* Patient-doctor
    relationships, strategies in; GPs,
    strategies to manage uncertainty/
    anxiety
Stress   91, 96
Stroke   9
Surgery
  fetal transplants   7
  stereotactic   65
Survey techniques   113
Survival strategies   30
'Switching off'   30-31

Terminal care   70, 109
Time   72-75, 77-79, 104, 112, 116, 123, 125
  attitudes to   73
  flexible approaches to   81
  focus on the present   45, 89
  management of   89
  past and future   89
  restructuring and reshaping of
    perspectives of   45, 87-89
Training and medical education   109-111
Tremor   59
Typicality   113

Uncertainty   4-5, 41-42, 54, 62-63
  accepting of   73
  additional   56, 60
  and Avoiders   26
  clarification of   28
  clinical   6, 44, 50
  concept of   xi, 5-6
  functional, use of   19-20
  and hospital physicians   5
  information and   11-40, 103-105
  management of   11, 21, 24, 30, 65-66, 82
    by GPs, *see* GPs, strategies to
    manage uncertainty/anxiety
    and closed policies concerning   24
    and flexible policies
    concerning   24
  neutralizing of   50
  and non-disclosures of
    information   11
  and partial disclosure of

information   11
restricting to manageable levels   52,
        81
and Seekers   26
sharing of, with patients   17-18, 68-
        82
strategies adopted by patients, *see*
        Patient-doctor relationships
and Weavers   26
see also under Patients, management
        of
Unease   79

Unpredictability, in prognosis and
        treatment   2
Unpredictable mood swings   9

Weavers   26, 28-31, 55, 66
'What patients can cope with'   17-19
Wheelchairs, as a focus for
        dependence   84
'Whole person'
    patient as a   94
    see also Individualized care